The Head and Neck Cancer Patient: Perioperative Care and Assessment

Editors

ZVONIMIR L. MILAS
THOMAS D. SHELLENBERGER

ORAL AND MAXILLOFACIAL SURGERY CLINICS OF NORTH AMERICA

www.oralmaxsurgery.theclinics.com

Consulting Editor
RUI P. FERNANDES

November 2018 • Volume 30 • Number 4

ELSEVIER

1600 John F. Kennedy Boulevard • Suite 1800 • Philadelphia, Pennsylvania, 19103-2899

http://www.oralmaxsurgery.theclinics.com

ORAL AND MAXILLOFACIAL SURGERY CLINICS OF NORTH AMERICA Volume 30, Number 4
November 2018 ISSN 1042-3699, ISBN-13: 978-0-323-64171-5

Editor: John Vassallo; j.vassallo@elsevier.com
Developmental Editor: Laura Fisher

Oral and Maxillofacial Surgery Clinics of North America (ISSN 1042-3699) is published quarterly by Elsevier Inc., 360 Park Avenue South, New York, NY 10010-1710. Months of issue are February, May, August, and November. Business and Editorial Offices: 1600 John F. Kennedy Blvd., Suite 1800, Philadelphia, PA 19103-2899. Periodicals postage paid at New York, NY and additional mailing offices. Subscription prices are $393.00 per year for US individuals, $686.00 per year for US institutions, $100.00 per year for US students and residents, $464.00 per year for Canadian individuals, $822.00 per year for Canadian institutions, $520.00 per year for international individuals, $822.00 per year for international institutions and $235.00 per year for Canadian and foreign students/residents. To receive student/resident rate, orders must be accompanied by name or affiliated institution, date of term, and the *signature* of program/residency coordinator on institution letterhead. Orders will be billed at individual rate until proof of status is received. Foreign air speed delivery is included in all *Clinics* subscription prices. All prices are subject to change without notice. **POSTMASTER:** Send address changes to *Oral and Maxillofacial Surgery Clinics of North America,* Elsevier Periodicals **Customer Service, 11830 Westline Industrial Drive, St. Louis, MO 63146. Tel: 1-800-654-2452 (U.S. and Canada); 314-447-8871 (outside U.S. and Canada). Fax: 314-447-8029. E-mail: journals customerservice-usa@elsevier.com (for print support); journalsonlinesupport-usa@elsevier.com (for online support)**.

Reprints. For copies of 100 or more, of articles in this publication, please contact the Commercial Reprints Department, Elsevier Inc., 360 Park Avenue South, New York, NY 10010-1710. Tel.: 212-633-3874; Fax: 212-633-3820; Email: reprints@elsevier.com.

Oral and Maxillofacial Surgery Clinics of North America is covered in *MEDLINE/PubMed* (*Index Medicus*), *Science Citation Index Expanded (SciSearch®)*, *Journal Citation Reports/Science Edition*, and *Current Contents®/Clinical Medicine*.

Contributors

CONSULTING EDITOR

RUI P. FERNANDES, MD, DMD, FACS, FRCS(Ed)
Clinical Professor and Chief, Division of Head and Neck Surgery, Departments of Oral and Maxillofacial Surgery, Neurosurgery, and Orthopaedic Surgery & Rehabilitation, University of Florida Health Science Center, University of Florida College of Medicine, Jacksonville, FL, USA

EDITORS

ZVONIMIR L. MILAS, MD, FACS
Associate Professor and Director, Head and Neck Cancer Center, Division of Surgical Oncology, Levine Cancer Institute, Atrium Healthcare, Charlotte, North Carolina, USA

THOMAS D. SHELLENBERGER, DMD, MD, FACS
Head and Neck Surgical Oncologist, Division of Surgical Oncology, Banner MD Anderson Cancer Center, Gilbert, Arizona, USA; Adjunct Assistant Professor, Department of Head and Neck Surgery, The University of Texas MD Anderson Cancer Center, Houston, Texas, USA

AUTHORS

ALI ALIAS, B.Sc
M.Sc.(A) Candidate, MD, CM Candidate, Faculty of Medicine, McGill University, Montreal, Quebec, Canada

LONI C. ARRESE, PhD
Assistant Professor, Department of Otolaryngology–Head and Neck Surgery, The Ohio State University, Columbus, Ohio, USA

NAFI AYGUN, MD
Division of Neuroradiology, Johns Hopkins University, School of Medicine, Baltimore, Maryland, USA

AARON H. BAER, MD
Section of Neuroradiology, Charlotte Radiology, Charlotte, North Carolina, USA

LAUREN C. CAPOZZI, MD, PhD
Division of Physical Medicine and Rehabilitation and Faculty of Medicine, Cumming School of Medicine, Foothills Medical Centre, Alberta, Canada

AMY Y. CHEN, MD, MPH
Department of Otolaryngology–Head and Neck Surgery, Emory University School of Medicine, Atlanta, Georgia, USA

NATASHA COHEN, MD, MSc, FRCSC
Department of Otolaryngology–Head and Neck Surgery, Emory University School of Medicine, Atlanta, Georgia, USA

NAOMI D. DOLGOY, OT
PhD Candidate, Faculty of Rehabilitation Medicine, University of Alberta, Edmonton, Alberta, Canada

JOEL EPSTEIN, DMD, MSD, FRCD(C), FDS RCS(Edin)
Consulting Staff, Division of Otolaryngology and Head and Neck Surgery, City of Hope, Duarte, California, USA

DONALD GREGORY FARWELL, MD
Professor and Chair, Department of Otolaryngology–Head and Neck Surgery, The UC Davis School of Medicine, Sacramento, California, USA

STACEY FEDEWA, PhD
American Cancer Society, Atlanta, Georgia, USA

AMARBIR GILL, MD
Resident Physician, Department of Otolaryngology–Head and Neck Surgery, UC Davis School of Medicine, Sacramento, California, USA

STEVEN P. HAUG, DDS, MSD, FACP
Professor, Department of Prosthodontics, Indiana University School of Dentistry, Indianapolis, Indiana, USA

MELISSA HENRY, PhD
Assistant Professor, Department of Oncology, Faculty of Medicine, McGill University, FRQS Clinician-Scientist, Jewish General Hospital, Montreal, Quebec, Canada

KATHERINE A. HUTCHESON, PhD
Associate Professor, Department of Head and Neck Surgery, The University of Texas MD Anderson Cancer Center, Houston, Texas, USA

MARYAM JESSRI, DDS, PhD
Chief Resident, Division of Oral Medicine and Dentistry, Brigham and Women's Hospital, Boston, Massachusetts, USA

JOSHUA E. LUBEK, MD, DDS, FACS
Fellowship Director, Oral–Head and Neck Surgery/Microvascular Surgery, Associate Professor, Department of Oral and Maxillofacial Surgery, University of Maryland, Baltimore, Maryland, USA

MARGARET L. McNEELY, PT, PhD
Associate Professor, Faculty of Rehabilitation Medicine, University of Alberta, Cross Cancer Institute, Edmonton, Alberta, Canada

MICHAEL G. MOORE, MD
Director of Head and Neck Surgery, Associate Professor, Department of Otolaryngology– Head and Neck Surgery, UC Davis School of Medicine, Sacramento, California, USA

KAMOLPHOB PHASUK, DDS, MS, FACP
Clinical Assistant Professor, Department of Prosthodontics, Indiana University School of Dentistry, Indianapolis, Indiana, USA

DANIEL P. SEEBURG, MD, PhD
Section of Neuroradiology, Charlotte Radiology, Charlotte, North Carolina, USA

THOMAS D. SHELLENBERGER, DMD, MD, FACS
Head and Neck Surgical Oncologist, Division of Surgical Oncology, Banner MD Anderson Cancer Center, Gilbert, Arizona, USA; Adjunct Assistant Professor, Department of Head and Neck Surgery, The University of Texas MD Anderson Cancer Center, Houston, Texas, USA

HERVE Y. SROUSSI, DMD, PhD
Associate Surgeon, Division of Oral Medicine and Dentistry, Brigham and Women's Hospital, Dana-Farber Cancer Institute, Boston, Massachusetts, USA

RANDAL S. WEBER, MD
Chief Patient Experience Officer, Division of Ofc/EVP, Physician-in-Chief, John Brooks Williams and Elizabeth Williams Distinguished University Chair in Cancer Medicine, Professor, Department of Head and Neck Surgery, Division of Surgery, The University of Texas MD Anderson Cancer Center, Houston, Texas, USA

Contents

Head and neck malignancies comprise a heterogeneous group of malignancies that cause significant morbidity to those affected. These malignancies are associated with specific risk factors and exposures, some of which affect prognosis. The most common risk factors for developing head and neck cancers are tobacco and alcohol use. Marijuana and e-cigarettes, occupational exposures, and use of topical substances have also been linked to head and neck cancers. Human papilloma virus has been associated with oropharyngeal cancer. Measures such as oral hygiene, screening, smoking cessation, and vaccination have been taken to decrease the incidence and morbidity of head and neck cancers.

This article provides a framework for speech-language pathology services to optimize functional outcomes of patients with oral cavity and oropharyngeal cancers. Key principles include (1) a proactive rehabilitation model that minimizes intervals of disuse or inactivity of speech and swallowing systems, (2) standardized evaluation paradigms that combine objective instrumental assessments with patient-reported outcome measures, and (3) systematic methods for surveillance and intensive rehabilitation for late dysphagia.

Recovery after major head and neck cancer surgery is a complex process. These patients frequently suffer from malnutrition, in addition to perioperative sequelae such as pain, wound infections, venous thromboembolism (VTE), and pneumonia. The authors provide a contemporary evidence-based approach to common aspects of perioperative care to guide the clinician in the optimal management of patients. Particular emphasis is placed on the preoperative education of patients and the identification and management of malnutrition around the time of surgery. This article discusses recommendations for perioperative antibiotics, pain management, and prophylaxis against VTE and pneumonia in this patient population.

In this article, the authors summarize the latest imaging methods and recommendations for each of the various steps in managing patients with head and neck cancer, from staging of disease to posttreatment surveillance. Because staging of head and neck cancers is different for various subsites of the head and neck, imaging is discussed separately for each. A separate discussion of imaging of perineural spread, occult primary tumors, and lymph nodes is followed by a discussion of paradigms for surveillance imaging in the posttreatment neck.

The multidisciplinary team planning conference is critical in the evaluation and management of patients with head and neck cancer. The management is complex and dictates the care of a multidisciplinary team for optimal results. First, the head and neck multidisciplinary team ensures the complete evaluation of patients before beginning treatment. Second, the team improves the accuracy of diagnosis and staging on which to base the most appropriate treatment. Third, the team improves the outcomes of treatment by appealing to the best available evidence, by following clinical practice guidelines and treatment algorithms and by engaging in clinical research trials.

Patients undergoing treatment of head and neck cancer risk developing significant acute and chronic changes that affect the hard and soft tissue of the oral cavity and the head and neck region. This article discusses considerations and recommendations for patients before, during, and after treatment of head and neck cancer. The objective of these recommendations is to maintain oral health, compensate for treatment- and disease-associated morbidities, and improve quality of life. To achieve this objective, treatment of head and neck cancer must include an oral evaluation and management plan well integrated within the overall oncologic treatment plan from the initiation of therapy.

Ongoing genetic and epigenetic research involving DNA methylation, salivary biomarkers, wild-type p53 tumor suppressor gene proteins, and HPV oncogenes are being directed at identification and treatment of dysplastic and malignant squamous cell mucosal lesions. Research is being conducted to improve immunotherapy drug response rates by increasing the amount of inflammation within the tumor microenvironment. Ongoing research is focused on the application of the antidiabetic drug metformin for the prevention and management of oral squamous cell dysplastic lesions. Professional and nonprofit cancer support organizations are essential for furthering education and research within the area of head and neck cancer.

Head and neck cancer and associated treatments can have debilitating effects on patient physical function and quality of life. The American Cancer Society's Head and Neck Cancer Survivorship Care Guidelines recommend that all patients receive an assessment after their treatment to address complications that may affect long-term recovery and function. Evidence supports the role of physical activity, exercise, physical therapy, and occupational therapy to decrease symptom burden after treatment and improve strength, endurance, and function. Physical therapy can play an important role in optimizing jaw, neck, and shoulder function, and occupational therapy can optimize return to work.

Maxillofacial Prosthetics 487

Kamolphob Phasuk and Steven P. Haug

The treatment of head and neck cancers requires a team approach. Maxillofacial prosthetics and oncologic dentistry are involved in many phases of the treatment. After the cancer ablation surgery, if surgical reconstruction cannot completely restore the surgical defect site, maxillofacial prostheses play an important role in rehabilitating the patient's mastication, swallowing, and speech. For patients undergoing chemoradiation therapy, the outcome is enhanced by jaw positioning stent and fluoride carrier mouthpiece. This perioperative care by maxillofacial prosthetics improves the posttreatment outcomes and the patient's quality of life.

Psychosocial Effects of Head and Neck Cancer 499

Ali Alias and Melissa Henry

Head and neck cancer is known to be both physically and psychologically challenging. This article summarizes the literature on the psychosocial effects of head and neck cancer by distinguishing features in the preoperative and postoperative periods. It outlines the importance of an integrated collaborative care approach in clinics as well as areas worthy of further program development.

ORAL AND MAXILLOFACIAL SURGERY CLINICS OF NORTH AMERICA

SERIES OF RELATED INTEREST

Atlas of the Oral and Maxillofacial Surgery Clinics
www.oralmaxsurgeryatlas.theclinics.com

Dental Clinics
www.dental.theclinics.com

THE CLINICS ARE NOW AVAILABLE ONLINE!
Access your subscription at:
www.theclinics.com

Preface
Getting It Right from the Start

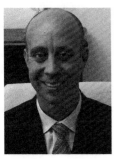
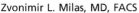
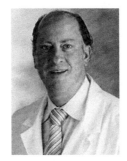

Zvonimir L. Milas, MD, FACS   Thomas D. Shellenberger, DMD, MD, FACS
Editors

In the first of two issues that focus on the patient with head and neck cancer, we sharpen our perspective on the initial assessment and planning of care. Patients with head and neck cancer require a true multidisciplinary team approach from the beginning where appropriate imaging, medical and dental evaluation, functional and nutritional assessment, and discussion of treatment goals are critical to guiding the patient in treatment. Our aim to get it right from the start sets the stage for defining these goals of treatment and thereby locks in the best chances for achieving those goals that are most important to our patients. This first issue offers a synthesis of the best, current evidence on which to base care from initial presentation, through diagnosis and staging, and on to the execution of a plan of care. All light is shed from the vantage points of key members of a spectrum of health care providers devoted to patients with head and neck cancer.

As technological advances break barriers of past decades and open new doors to improving the outcomes of patients with head and neck cancer, the response to the call brings an urgency like never before. Indeed, all members of the diverse multidisciplinary head and neck team are currently poised to impact the care of patients with head and neck cancer like never before. And while the disease remains among the most devastating, the resolve of dedicated clinicians continues to meet these challenges like never

before. Yet, as the availability of treatment options expands at an alarming rate, the greatest priorities for clinicians remain: to come to know our patients, to teach our patients by sharing our knowledge, and to join our patients in the battle of fighting their disease. Along the way, our patients come to know themselves better and find deep within them a capacity they never knew could emerge.

We hope readers of the *Oral and Maxillofacial Surgery Clinics of North America* will gain new insight and find practical perspectives to benefit their patients from each of the articles submitted by our contributors. The function of the head and neck multidisciplinary team and the tumor board is discussed. The most current epidemiologic data of head and neck cancer are interpreted. And the critical contribution of speech pathology, pretreatment pathways, and nutritional optimization is reviewed. The current status and optimal use of diagnostic imaging, and perioperative dental assessment, are summarized. In addition, the current focus of translational research in head and neck cancer is distilled. Finally, the role of prehabilitation and rehabilitation by physical and occupational therapy and by maxillofacial prosthetics is highlighted. While by no means comprehensive, we hope nonetheless the issue will refine clinical judgment and decision making, enhance the knowledge of surgical and oncologic principles, and inspire a deeper sense of purpose in the care of patients with head and neck cancer.

Oral Maxillofacial Surg Clin N Am 30 (2018) ix–x
https://doi.org/10.1016/j.coms.2018.08.001
1042-3699/18/© 2018 Published by Elsevier Inc.

We are indebted to the vast knowledge, skills, and dedication of the many clinicians and researchers who have committed much time and effort to their contributions of this issue. We also owe an incredible debt of gratitude to our patients to whom our work serves as a monument. And last, without the tireless support of our families, none of our efforts can bear fruit.

Zvonimir L. Milas, MD, FACS
Head and Neck Cancer Center
Division of Surgical Oncology
Atrium Healthcare
Levine Cancer Institute, Suite 3300
1021 Morehead Medical Drive
Charlotte, NC 28204, USA

Thomas D. Shellenberger, DMD, MD, FACS
Division of Surgical Oncology
Banner MD Anderson Cancer Center
2946 E Banner Gateway Drive, Suite 450
Gilbert, AZ 85234, USA

Department of Head and Neck Surgery
The University of Texas MD Anderson
Cancer Center
Houston, TX, USA

E-mail addresses:
Zvonimir.Milas@carolinashealthcare.org
(Z.L. Milas)
thomas.shellenberger@bannerhealth.com
(T.D. Shellenberger)

Epidemiology and Demographics of the Head and Neck Cancer Population

Natasha Cohen, MD, MSc, FRCSC[a], Stacey Fedewa, PhD[b],
Amy Y. Chen, MD, MPH[a],*

KEYWORDS

• Risk factors • Epidemiology • Cancer • HPV • Head and neck

KEY POINTS

• Head and neck malignancies affect the oral cavity, pharynx, larynx, salivary glands, and sinonasal cavities.
• Risk factors for head and neck malignancies vary based on subsites. These include tobacco smoke exposure, alcohol use, HPV, marijuana, and smokeless tobacco.
• The incidence of head and neck cancers is mostly declining because of successful public health smoking cessation campaigns with the exception of HPV-related malignancies.
• Demographic factors are linked to increased incidence, advanced stage at presentation, and poor prognosis.
• Early detection can help prevent significant functional and cosmetic morbidity and mortality. To date, no evidence-based screening protocols have been validated.

INTRODUCTION

Malignancies of the head and neck affect a variety of anatomic subsites, including the skin, oral cavity, oropharynx, nasopharynx, hypopharynx, larynx, paranasal sinuses, and salivary glands. Although malignancies of the epithelial origin, namely squamous cell carcinoma, are most common, neoplasms of mesenchymal, neural, and other cellular origins do occur. The use of tobacco and alcohol have been long recognized as major risk factors for the development of squamous cell carcinoma in the head and neck. Human papilloma virus (HPV) has also been found to be a major contributor to the development of oropharyngeal squamous cell carcinoma.[1] Other risk factors include genetics, toxic exposures, diet, and environmental factors.

This article discusses the epidemiology of head and neck cancer (HNC), including risk factors, incidence, prognosis, survival, and health advocacy measures to be considered when caring for patients with HNC.

EPIDEMIOLOGY OF HEAD AND NECK CANCER

HNC is a heterogeneous entity, comprising malignancies arising above the thoracic inlet and below the level of the skull base. According to the definition from the American Joint Committee on Cancer, head and neck oncology encompasses malignancies arising from mucosal surfaces from the oral cavity, pharynx, larynx, and paranasal sinuses, and cancers originating from major and minor salivary glands.[2] Much of the

Disclosure: The authors have nothing to disclose.
[a] Department of Otolaryngology–Head and Neck Surgery, Emory University School of Medicine, 550 Peachtree Street. MOT 1135, Atlanta, GA 30308, USA; [b] American Cancer Society, 250 Williams Street. NW, Atlanta, GA 30303, USA
* Corresponding author.
E-mail address: achen@emory.edu

Oral Maxillofacial Surg Clin N Am 30 (2018) 381–395
https://doi.org/10.1016/j.coms.2018.06.001
1042-3699/18/Published by Elsevier Inc.

data regarding risk factors for HNC presented in this article are derived from a multicenter, international endeavor known as the International Head and Neck Cancer Epidemiology Consortium (INHANCE), which pooled the data collected from 35 epidemiologic studies of HNC. The aggregate data were collected from case-control studies and case series comparing a total of 25,000 patients and 37,100 control subjects from the Unites States, Europe, Brazil, Latin America, and Asia, and this aggregate data was used to inform epidemiologic conclusions with the statistical power needed to confidently understand HNC risk.[3]

Oral Cavity and Pharynx

According to the Surveillance, Epidemiology, and End Results Program database, the prevalence of oral cavity and pharyngeal cancer (OCPC) in the United States in 2014 was 340,902.[4] Based on data collected between 2010 and 2014, the number of new cases or incidence of OCPC for women and men was 11.2/100,000.[4] Moreover, men were overall more likely to be diagnosed with these malignancies with 16.9 new cases out of 100,000 people, compared with 6.2/100,000 new cases for women. The rate of death for OCPC was similarly found to be increased in men compared with women (overall, 2.5 per 100,000; men, 3.8 per 100,000; women, 1.3 per 100 000), but interestingly black men were found to have the highest rate of death at 5.0 per 100,000. The American

Cancer Society estimates that in 2017 the number of new OCPC diagnosed will be 49,670 (35,720 men, 13,950 women), and 9700 deaths will occur as a result of OCPC (7000 men, 2700 women).[5] These estimates make OCPC the ninth most commonly diagnosed cancer in men, comprising 4% of all new cancer cases diagnosed in men. In fact, according to data collected between 2009 and 2013, men are diagnosed 2.7 times more frequently with and die 2.8 times more often of OCPC than women.[5] Overall 5-year survival for all OCPC was 64.7% based on 2007 to 2013 data.[4]

The incidence of OCPC has been rising on average by 0.6% per year for the last decade, with the incidence of oropharyngeal and tonsillar cancers increasing on average by 2.9% per year (**Fig. 1**). This is largely driven by a well-recognized increased prevalence of HPV-related malignancies, which mainly affect the oropharynx. In fact, Surveillance, Epidemiology, and End Results Program data show that between 2005 and 2014, the incidence of malignancies associated with HPV infections, such as those of the tonsil, oropharynx, other oral cavity, and oropharynx and tongue cancers have increased by 3%, 2.3%, 3.9%, and 1.7% per year, respectively, whereas the incidence of malignancies associated with traditional HNC risk factors (eg, tobacco, alcohol), such as cancers of the gums and other oral cavity, floor of mouth, and hypopharynx, have decreased by 0.1%, 3.0%, and 2.5% per year, respectively, over that same period of time.[6] Moreover, HPV-positive malignancies are

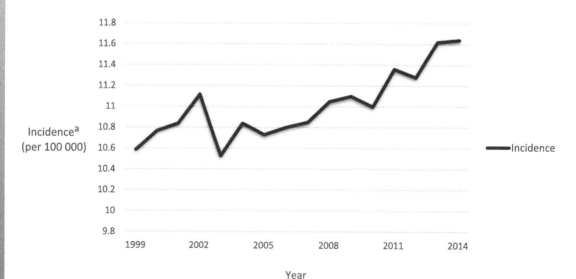

Fig. 1. US incidence of oral cavity and pharyngeal cancer. [a] Age- and delay-adjusted incidence rate per year. (*Data from* Howlader NNA, Krapcho M, Miller D, et al. SEER cancer statistics review, 1975-2014. 2017. Available at: https://seer.cancer.gov/csr/1975_2014/.)

well-recognized to be more sensitive to treatment and this has been evident in trends for mortality, where despite an increased incidence, malignancies of the tongue and other oral cavity and oropharyngeal site have seen a decrease in mortality of 0.1% and 2.2% per year, respectively. Moreover, despite their dramatic increase in incidence (3% per year), the mortality has only increased by 1.7%.[6]

Larynx

When considered independently, laryngeal cancer is an uncommon disease, with an incidence of 3.1 in 100,000, which translates to 13,360 new cases projected to be diagnosed in the United States in 2017.[7] It accounts for 0.8% of new cancer diagnoses and is the 20th most common malignancy diagnosed in the United States.[7] Moreover, unlike OCPC, the rate of laryngeal cancer has been steadily decreasing by 2.3% per year from 2005 to 2014. Men are more likely to develop laryngeal cancer than women, with a respective incidence of 4.1 compared with 0.9 per 100,000 (**Fig. 2**).[6] Overall survival for laryngeal cancer is comparable with other HNC, with a 5-year survival of 60.7% for all stages.[6]

Laryngeal cancer is most commonly associated with tobacco and alcohol intake. Based on data from INHANCE consortium, the risk of developing laryngeal cancer in nondrinkers with any amount of cigarette smoking is significantly increased compared with nonsmokers (odds ratio [OR], 6.84; 95% confidence interval [CI], 4.25–11.01).[8] There is a strong dose-dependent relationship between smoking and laryngeal cancer, with an increased risk found for increased quantity of cigarettes smoked per day and the number of years smoked.[8] However, in nonsmokers, the risk of laryngeal cancer for subjects who reported any

alcohol use compared with those who reported no alcohol use was not significant (OR, 1.21; 95% CI, 0.82–1.79), and a statistically significant increase in laryngeal cancer risk was only shown in those who drank five or more drinks per day.[8] In fact, alcohol use alone has not been strongly associated with laryngeal cancer, with multiple studies showing no association regardless of dose and exposure length.[9,10] However, evidence suggests that there is an increased risk of alcohol intake for developing cancer of the supraglottis compared with other laryngeal subsites.[10,11] Moreover, when combining the use of alcohol to cigarette smoking, a synergistic multiplicative risk exists for developing laryngeal cancer, with an OR ranging from 8.0 (95% CI, 2.0–22.80) for the lightest level of smoking and drinking, to 177.2 (95% CI, 65.0–483.3) for the heaviest level of smoking and drinking.[11]

Major and Minor Salivary Gland

Salivary gland malignancies comprise a heterogeneous group of malignancies histologically and pathophysiologically. Anatomically, the major salivary glands refer to the parotid, submandibular, and sublingual glands, whereas minor salivary glands are millimetric structures. The upper aerodigestive tract contains between 450 and 750 minor salivary glands.[12] Malignancies of the major and minor salivary glands are uncommon, with an incidence of 1.3 in 100,000, representing less than 9% of HNC,[6] and an overall 5-year survival of 71.9%.[6] Most salivary gland malignancies present in the parotid glands.[12] Unlike other subsites of the head and neck where epithelially derived malignancies, such as squamous cell carcinoma, are most common, the salivary glands are complex units comprised of various cell types, leading to a diverse set of malignancies arising from these

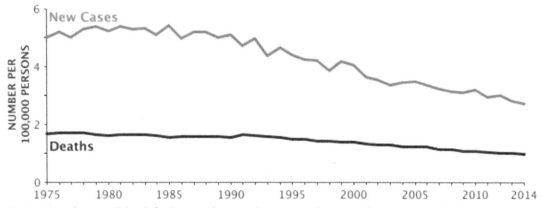

Fig. 2. US incidence and death for laryngeal cancer. (*From* Surveillance, Epidemiology, and End Results program. SEER cancer stat facts: laryngeal cancer. Available at: http://seer.cancer.gov/statfacts/html/laryn.html.)

glands each with different biologic behaviors and prognoses. Moreover, the superficial parotid gland contains lymph nodes that drain the skin from the frontotemporal scalp, face, and ear and these malignancies can extend into the deep lobe because of the absence of a fibrous capsule separating the superficial and deep parotid lobes.[13]

Few studies address the epidemiology of salivary gland malignancies by subtypes. Further complicating matters, the classification guidelines for salivary gland tumors has changed many times over the past few decades. Much of the knowledge about the incidence of salivary gland tumors has been extrapolated from the landmark retrospective study by Spiro and colleagues, published in 1986.[14] A more recent study by Boukheris and coworkers[15] reassessed this topic using the World Health Organization 2005 classification. The study reported the most commonly diagnosed major salivary malignancies were mucoepidermoid carcinoma (2.85 per 1,000,000 person-years), followed by squamous cell carcinoma (1.83 per 1,000,000 person-years), acinic cells carcinoma (1.38 per 1,000,000 person-years), adenoid cystic carcinoma (1.30 per 1,000,000 person-years) and adenocarcinoma not otherwise specified (1.22 per 1,000,000 person-years).[15] The incidence of other histologic types of salivary gland malignancies had an incidence rate less than 1 case per 1,000,000 person-years, for carcinoma ex-pleomorphic, epithelial-myoepithelial carcinoma, lymphoepithelial carcinoma, salivary duct carcinoma, basal cell carcinoma, oncocyctic carcinoma, and other even rarer subtypes.[15] The authors noted that because primary squamous cell carcinoma of major salivary glands is rare, such tumors could have been misclassified in their series.

Considering gender, men are 50% more likely than women to develop a salivary gland malignancy.[15] Unlike other HNC, salivary gland tumors are not strongly linked to tobacco and alcohol use. One notable exception, the incidence of papillary cystadenoma lymphomatosum or Warthin tumor is strongly associated with smoking.[16] Studies have shown that exposure to ionizing radiation, such as a nuclear event,[17,18] dental radiographs,[19,20] external beam radiotherapy,[21] or iodine 131 treatment,[22,23] increases the risk of developing benign and malignant tumors of the salivary glands. Other risk factors for malignant salivary tumors include early menarche,[24] and exposure to silica dust,[25] kerosene,[25] nickel, chromium, asbestos, and cement dust.[26]

Nasal Cavity and Paranasal Sinuses

Sinonasal malignancies are a rare entity, accounting for less than 1% of all malignancies and less than 5%

of HNC,[6] with an incidence of 0.556 per 100,000.[27] Sinonasal malignancies occur most commonly in the nasal cavity (43.9% of all sinonasal malignancies), followed by the maxillary sinuses (35.9%), ethmoid sinuses (9.5%), sphenoid sinuses (3.3%), and frontal sinuses (1.1%).[27] Sinonasal cancers occur almost twice as commonly in men than in women (1.8:1) and most malignancies derived from epithelial lining (squamous cell carcinoma 51.6% of sinonasal malignancies, adenocarcinoma 12.6%, esthesioneuroblastoma 6.3%, adenoid cystic carcinoma 6.2%) with the remaining histopathologic tumors comprising of melanoma (6.6%), sinonasal undifferentiated carcinoma (3.1%), and other (13.7%).[27] Survival rates vary based on the type of cancer, but overall, sinonasal cancer presents at advanced stages and carries a poor prognosis with an overall 5-year survival ranging between 30% and 40%.[28]

Sinonasal malignancies have most commonly been associated with occupational exposures, especially wood working,[29,30] which is associated with an increase in overall sinonasal malignancies (OR, 2.6; 95% CI, 2.1–3.3 for all histologic sinonasal cancers) and even more strongly associated with the development of adenocarcinoma (OR, 18; 95% CI, 12–28).[31] Among different types of wood workers, furniture workers were more likely to develop a sinonasal malignancy than carpenters (**Table 1**). Among wood workers, women were more likely to develop sinonasal cancers than men (OR, 3.4; 95% CI, 1.1–11). Other exposures that have been linked to developing sinonasal malignancies include formaldehyde[32,33]; asbestos[33]; textile dust[33]; metal industries,[34] such as aluminum,[35] copper and nickel,[36] and canning[34]; farming[34]; cocoa and chocolate production[34]; sugar confectionery[34]; and exposure to leather dust and mineral oils.[37]

Table 1		
Sinonasal cancers in wood workers by histology		
	All Histology[a]	**Adenocarcinoma[a]**
All wood workers	2.6 (2.1–3.3)	18 (12–28)
Furniture workers	2.4 (1.2–5.1)	29 (17–51)
Carpenters	1.6 (0.8–3.2)	18 (11–30)

[a] Results expressed as odds ratio (95% confidence interval).
Data from Gordon I, Boffetta P, Demers PA. A case study comparing a meta-analysis and a pooled analysis of studies of sinonasal cancer among wood workers. Epidemiology 1998;9(5):518–24.

Other risk factors for sinonasal cancers include smoking, which is associated with an increased risk of squamous cell carcinoma (OR, 1.72; 95% CI, 1.16–2.56)[38] but not adenocarcinoma.[39] HPV-DNA has been identified in some sinonasal cancers, particularly in nonkeratinizing squamous cell cancers.[40] This is not surprising because SCC of the nasal cavity has been associated with malignant degeneration of schneiderian papillomas (eg, inverting papilloma),[41] which have also been linked to HPV infection. In fact, a meta-analysis of 76 studies examining 1956 papillomas found that 38.8% of these tested positive for HPV.[42]

RISK FACTORS FOR HEAD AND NECK CANCER
Tobacco

Tobacco use is the leading cause of preventable death in the world[43] and tobacco smoking alone is the leading cause of cancer and cancer-related deaths worldwide.[44] Within the head and neck it has been conclusively shown to directly cause oral cavity, laryngeal, and pharyngeal cancer.[45] The International Agency for Research on Cancer (IARC) has classified tobacco smoking, second-hand smoking, and smokeless tobacco (SLT) as a group 1 carcinogen for HNCs,[46] where group 1 carcinogens are defined as agents with sufficient evidence of carcinogenicity to humans.[47] In developed countries, most inhaled or "mainstream" tobacco smoke comes from use of manufactured cigarettes. These burn at a high temperature and generate smoke that contains more than 7000 chemical compounds including carcinogens and toxins.[48] Similarly, pipes, cigars, and water pipes deliver smoke with a similar composition and therefore toxicity.[44,48]

Although tobacco smoke contains a range of group 1 carcinogens, including benzene, arsenic, polonium-210, nickel compounds, and beryllium,[44] research has focused on the link of tobacco-specific N-nitrosamines, especially N-nitrosonornicotine and 4-(N-nitrosomethylamino)-1-(3-pyridyl)-1-butanone, because of their established carcinogenicity. The latter are formed during the curing process and are especially high in dark tobacco. It is therefore not surprising that dark tobacco has been associated with increased risk of developing head and neck squamous cell carcinoma (HNSCC) compared with blonde tobacco.[49] The chemical composition, psychoactive effect, and flavor are dependent on plant genetics, weather conditions, curing, and agricultural practices, and is classified by the color of the resultant tobacco product. Commercially produced cigarettes contain proprietary mixtures of tobacco types, and there are geographic variations of tobacco types use. Dark tobacco is found in higher proportions in cigarettes sold in Europe and South America, and in chewing tobacco, whereas blond or light tobacco is found predominantly in cigarettes sold in the United States and Canada.[50] Filtered cigarettes decrease the exposure to the aforementioned carcinogens and only confer a 1.5 times increased risk of HNSCC compared with nonsmokers, whereas the risk with unfiltered cigarette use was 7.8 times higher than non-smokers.[51] Similarly, hand-rolled cigarettes confer a risk 8.7 times higher than nonsmokers of developing HNSCC.[51] Another compound that has been linked with an increased risk of cancer is tar, where higher tar contents has been shown to increase the risk of cancer.[52]

The risk of developing HNC posed by tobacco smoking is strongly dose-dependent, but exists even at low daily usage. Data from the INHANCE consortium shows that compared with non-smokers, any cigarette use increased the risk of HNC (0–3 cigarettes per day: OR, 1.52; 95% CI, 1.21–1.90), and use of 5 to 10 cigarettes daily more than doubles the risk of developing an HNC (overall OR, 2.6; 95% CI, 2.00–3.40).[53] Moreover, cigarette smoking presents an independent risk from alcohol; nondrinkers who smoked three to five cigarettes per day were more likely than those who did not smoke to develop HNC (OR, 2.14; 95% CI, 1.73–2.65). Excluding oropharyngeal cancers, which are often associated with HPV, demonstrated that smoking further increased the risk of nonoropharyngeal HNC, with daily use of 5 to 10 cigarettes conferring an OR of 2.98 (95% CI, 2.31–3.82).[53] Certain subsites, such as the larynx and hypopharynx, are more susceptible to lower daily exposure to cigarette smoke (**Table 2**). Moreover, the duration of exposure also significantly affects the risk of HNC. In fact, there was no statically significant increase in risk seen for the use of 5 to 10 cigarettes per day for less than 20 years, compared with daily use of three to five cigarettes for more than 20 years more than doubling the risk of HNC (20–30 years OR, 2.35; 95% CI, 1.52–3.65; more than 30 years OR, 2.89; 95% CI, 2.13–3.91). The highest risk for low daily average use was found for those smoking 5 to 10 cigarettes per day for more than 30 years (OR, 4.17; 95% CI, 3.54–4.90).[53]

Cigars/Pipes

Although cigar and pipe smoking are not as common as cigarette smoking, they can contain higher doses of carcinogens.[44] Wyss and coworkers[54] used data from the INHANCE consortium to assess the risk of cancer with pipe and cigar

Table 2
Head and neck cancer risk of average lifetime daily cigarette use

Average Lifetime Daily Cigarette Use	Odds Ratio (95% CI) by Head and Neck Subsite[a]				
	Overall	Oral Cavity	Hypopharynx	Oropharynx	Larynx
0–3[b]	1.52 (1.21–1.90)	1.48 (1.04–2.09)	2.43 (1.23–4.79)	1.57 (1.10–2.23)	2.68 (1.82–3.95)
3–5[b]	2.14 (1.73–2.65)	2.23 (1.45–3.42)	3.35 (1.78–6.29)	2.17 (1.53–3.06)	3.48 (2.40–5.05)
5–10[b]	2.60 (2.00–3.40)	2.18 (1.68–2.83)	4.38 (2.82–6.82)	2.85 (1.89–4.08)	5.21 (4.07–6.68)
11–20[c]	2.36 (1.60–3.47)	—	—	—	—
21–30[c]	3.58 (2.09–6.16)	—	—	—	—
31–40[c]	4.46 (2.54–7.83)	—	—	—	—
>40[c]	2.69 (1.21–5.98)	—	—	—	—

[a] Risk for smokers compared with nonsmokers.
[b] Data from Berthiller et al,[53] 2016.
[c] Data from Hashibe et al,[8] 2007.

Data from Berthiller J, Straif K, Agudo A, et al. Low frequency of cigarette smoking and the risk of head and neck cancer in the INHANCE consortium pooled analysis. Int J Epidemiol 2016;45(3):835–45; and Hashibe M, Brennan P, Benhamou S, et al. Alcohol drinking in never users of tobacco, cigarette smoking in never drinkers, and the risk of head and neck cancer: pooled analysis in the International Head and Neck Cancer Epidemiology Consortium. J Natl Cancer Inst 2007;99(10):777–89.

use. As compared with nonsmokers, the OR for developing HNSCC in cigar smokers was 2.54 (95% CI, 1.93–3.34), and 2.08 (95% CI, 1.54–3.45) in pipe smokers. They also noted a significant dose relationship for increased exposure to cigar and pipe smoking in patients who had never smoked cigarettes, but interestingly, the odds of developing HNSCC were not significantly higher in cigar and pipe users who also smoked cigarettes when compared with those who did not use any of the aforementioned products. When investigating the risk of cigar and pipe smoking by head and neck subsite, the laryngeal subsite exhibited the highest OR of cancer (6.31 for cigar and 3.53 for pipe), whereas the ORs for the other subsites were comparable regardless of the type of tobacco product. Other factors found to increase the risk of developing HNCs were age greater than 45 years and geographic location (Europe and South America was found to be at increased risk compared with North American smokers).

Smokeless Tobacco

SLT refers to formulations that are chewed, sucked or dissolved. It is known by many different names and formats including oral tobacco, chewing tobacco, spit, dip, and snuff.[55] It is estimated that in the United States, the prevalence of SLT use in adults is 2.3%,[56] which is comparable with 12th graders, of whom 2.8% report regular use.[57] SLT has been used as a harm-reduction method by substituting cigarette use for SLT because of evidence that cigarette smoking is

more addictive, produces a more severe withdrawal and higher rate of relapse compared with SLT,[58] and the absence of the risk conferred by second-hand smoke. Moreover, the lack of combustion reduces, but does not eliminate, the toxicity of tobacco.[59] SLT is known to cause leukoplakia and precancerous changes in the oral cavity and increases the risk of oral cancer 50-fold compared with nonusers.[60] In fact, similar to cigarette smoke, SLT contains tobacco-specific *N*-nitrosamines and these have been shown to cause oral cancer in in vivo rat models.[61] The risk of cancer varies based on the type of SLT used, with dry snuff producing the highest risk of oral cancer.[62]

Vaping

Vaping refers to the inhalation of vapor or steam produced by e-cigarettes or vaporizers from liquids that contain nicotine, flavorings, and a variety of other ingredients.[63,64] The popularity and use of vaping has dramatically increased in recent years,[65] in part because of the availability of a variety of flavors, which increases appeal to children and youth, and increased marketing and promotion of e-cigarettes as a healthier and more palatable alternative to traditional cigarette use.[66,67] It has also become regarded as an alternative and as a means for smoking cessation[68] because of the similarity of e-cigarettes to traditional cigarettes. The National Health Interview Survey began collecting e-cigarette usage data in 2014, therefore large-scale usage trends are not yet available. However, a report published from these data in

2015[65] showed that 3.7% of American adults were current users of e-cigarettes, with more than 20% of adults aged 18 to 24 having tried e-cigarettes, while use decreased with increasing age. The link between e-cigarettes and vaporizers to use by youth was also identified in high school students where the 30-day prevalence of vaping was more than twice that of regular cigarettes, and was calculated at 6.2% for 8th graders, 11% for 10th graders, and 13% for 12th graders.[66] Even more concerning was the finding that less than 22% of students in all grades perceived regular use of vaporizers as a "great risk,"[66] further demonstrating the benign perception of vaping. Moreover, a report from the Centers for Disease Control and Prevention indicated that between 2011 and 2016, use in high school children increased from 1.5% to 11.3%.[69] Despite the perception that the vapor from e-cigarettes does not cause harm, exposure of e-cigarette vapor with and without nicotine has been shown to be cytotoxic and induce DNA-strand breaks in epithelial cell lines in vitro.[70,71] As such, although previously unregulated, e-cigarettes and other electronic nicotine delivery systems have recently been addressed by the Food and Drug Administration, which has limited the sale of e-cigarettes and related products to customers aged 18 and older. In addition, as of August 2018 these products will be required to display a health warning.[72]

Although e-cigarettes have been used as smoking cessation adjuncts, there remains sparse evidence to support its use. A Cochrane review[73] has investigated the evidence supporting the use of e-cigarettes for smoking cessation. It identified three randomized controlled trials and 21 prospective cohort studies, and based on the evidence in the randomized controlled trials they concluded that there was no difference in successful tobacco abstinence between e-cigarettes and the nicotine patch[74] or placebo[74,75] (the third randomized controlled trial was not included in the analysis because of methodologic differences[57]). Nonetheless, e-cigarette use continues to grow, with a dramatic increase in prevalence of vaping in children and young adults. This is not surprising in light of evidence presented in a recent prospective cohort study that followed tobacco-naive young adults and showed that 47.7% of those who smoked e-cigarettes initiated smoking compared with 10.2% who did not (OR, 6.8; 95% CI, 1.7–28.3).[76] Because of disease lag time, e-cigarettes may not be conclusively linked to HNC for several years, but the evidence presented points toward e-cigarettes leading youth toward smoking cigarettes and therefore these should not continue to be portrayed as benign entities.

Marijuana

Marijuana is the most commonly used illicit drug in the world. Marijuana is made from the hemp plant or *Cannabis Sativa*, and confers a psychoactive effect to users because of its active compound delta-9-tetrahydrocannabinol.[77] The National Institute of Health (NIH) estimates the lifetime prevalence of marijuana or hashish use in 2016 was 44% for Americans ages 12 and older, with the highest prevalence reaching more than 50% in those aged 18 to 25.[78] The NIH also estimates that the lifetime prevalence of marijuana/hashish use in school-aged children is 13.5% for 8th graders, 30.7% for 10th graders, and 45% for 12th graders.[78] Marijuana is most commonly consumed through smoking, and therefore creates similar carcinogens to cigarette smoke, including nitrosamines and polycyclic aromatic hydrocarbons,[79] and contains more tar than tobacco.[80] Although marijuana's mutagenicity has been shown in vitro,[81] few studies have linked marijuana to carcinogenicity in humans.

A case-control study conducted at Memorial Sloan Kettering by Zheng and colleagues[82] showed a statistically significant increase in the OR of 2.6 for developing HNCs in marijuana users. They also found a significant dose-response for increased marijuana use and increased risk of cancer, and an increased risk for subjects ages younger than 55. However, this study was small, with 173 cases and 176 control subjects studied. Several studies[83–87] since then have investigated this question and have not found an increased risk of HNC in marijuana users, regardless of frequency or duration of use. Nonetheless, these studies have significant limitations ranging from recall bias,[85] underpowered sample sizes and various other methodologic limitations.[83,84,87] Another interesting study by Gillison and coworkers[88] investigated differences in HPV-positive and -negative HNSCC and found that HPV-16 positivity was strongly associated with a history of marijuana use, and an increasing odds ratio for HPV-16-positive HNSCC with increased intensity of use. Despite the lack of high-quality evidence linking marijuana to HNSCC, it remains biologically plausible for marijuana smoke to play a role in its pathophysiology. The legalization of marijuana is progressively being adopted across the United States, leading to increased use of a substance with an unclear risk of malignancy.[89,90] Prospective and randomized studies addressing the clinical applications and adverse effects of marijuana have been limited because illicit drugs cannot be approved for study by the Food and Drug Administration, which has led to the limited availability of systematically collected data regarding the impact of marijuana use.[91,92] The ongoing increase in legal marijuana use presents an opportunity to generate data that could elucidate the truth regarding the risk marijuana poses for developing HNCs.

Alcohol

Alcohol intake is a well establish risk factor for most subsites of the head and neck,[93] and esophageal and gastric cancers.[94] Alcohol has been classified as an upper aerodigestive tract carcinogen by the IARC since 1988,[95] specifically listing the oral cavity, oropharynx, hypopharynx, and larynx as head and neck sites susceptible to its toxicity. There is a growing body of evidence elucidating the direct relationship between the risk of HNSCC and alcohol intake. In fact, tumors arising in patients who are never-smokers with a history of alcohol intake have genetic alterations distinct from those found in smokers.[96] It is, however, difficult to isolate the role of alcohol from smoking because they are most often coexisting risk factors and therefore a confounder in statistical risk calculations. Traditionally, concomitant use of tobacco and alcohol confers a 35-fold increased risk of HNSCC, compared with five-fold for tobacco alone and nine-fold for alcohol alone.[97] Contemporary studies have further characterized this risk, such as Hashibe and colleagues,[8] where the authors conducted a pooled analysis of 15 case control studies. They found that nonsmoking participants who had a history of any alcohol intake compared with those who did not had an increase in risk of HNC. However, this same nonsmoking population showed an increased risk of HNC when consumption of alcohol increased. In fact, intake of three or more drinks a day doubled the risk of HNSCC compared with those who did not drink alcohol (OR, 2.04; 95% CI, 1.29–3.21). A subgroup analysis by head and neck subsite further revealed that the increased risk for pharyngeal cancer was conferred by only one to two drinks per day (OR, 1.66; 95% CI, 1.18–2.34), compared with five or more drinks per day for laryngeal cancer (OR, 2.98; 95% CI, 1.72–5.17).[8] Freedman and colleagues[9] looked at the population cohort from the NIH-AARP Diet and Health Study[98] and risk factors for HNCs and found that women were more susceptible to the carcinogenic effects of alcohol than their male counterparts, even when controlled for age and smoking status. Moreover, the dose-response relationship to increased alcohol intake more strongly correlated with an increased risk of cancer for women than men.

Human Papilloma Virus

HPV is a double-stranded DNA virus transmitted through direct contact and has more than 200 known serotypes, many of which cause benign epithelial lesions, such as the common wart.[99] However, certain high-risk subtypes of HPV are known to promote carcinogenesis, such as 16, 18, and 31, which have been shown to lead to the development of cervical, anogenital, and oropharyngeal cancer.[100] Based on National Health and Nutrition Examination Survey data from 2003 to 2006, the prevalence of HPV infection ranged from 32.9% to 53.8% between age groups, with the peak prevalence found among 20 to 24 year olds (data collected in women only but assumed to be the same in men)[101] making it the most common known sexually transmitted infection.[102] The natural history of HPV infection is characterized by spontaneous regression in 70% to 93% of cases over 1 to 2 years.[103,104] The mechanism by which HPV causes premalignant and malignant changes has been derived from knowledge acquired from cervical cancer research. Following sexual contact, HPV infects keratinocytes in the basal layer of squamous epithelium and replicates within their nucleus.[105] The HPV genome encodes for six early proteins (E1, E2, E4, E5, E6, E7) and two late proteins (L1, L2). Molecular studies show that in high-risk HPV serotypes, E6 and E7 behave as oncoproteins by binding the tumor-suppressor proteins p53 and pRB, respectively, and promoting their degradation,[106] resulting in genomic instability, unregulated cell-growth, and ultimately progression to malignancy.[107] As a tumor suppressor pRB inhibits the gene encoding p16. In the presence of a high-risk HPV infection, the absence of pRB leads to the overexpression of p16, which is detected with immunohistochemistry and has been use by pathologist as a surrogate marker for HPV in the setting of oropharyngeal cancer.[108]

The link between HPV and oropharyngeal cancer was first described in a study by Gillison and coworkers[109] in 2000. The study identified HPV in 25% of HNC specimens, but 62% of tonsil and tongue base tumors. The other subsites found to be positive for HPV were the larynx (19%), oral cavity (12%), and hypopharynx (10%). The most common HPV serotype found in these tumors was HPV16 (90%) followed by HPV33 (5%), HPV18 (2%), and HPV31 (2%) The authors also described important differences between HPV-positive and -negative tumors, such as smoking and alcohol exposure, which were lower in HPV-positive tumors, and markedly improved outcomes for patients with HPV-positive tumors (adjusted hazard ratio for death, 0.41; 95% CI, 0.2–0.88).[109] Since then, knowledge of HPV-positive head and neck disease has grown significantly, and its distinct molecular biology has been further characterized.

HPV-related HNSCC has been shown to display a specific histology, predominantly nonkeratinizing morphology[110] with a basaloid or poorly differentiated morphology.[111] This terminology is falling out of favor because it creates confusion since basaloid and poorly differentiated squamous cell carcinomas are a separate entity, and these histologic features are associated with significantly poorer prognosis in non-HPV-related cancers.[111,112] Patients with HPV-positive cancers are more likely to present with cervical lymphadenopathy with cystic degeneration than those with HPV-negative HNC,[113,114] but unlike HPV-negative tumors, nodal disease in HPV-positive HNC does not confer the same poor prognostic implication.[115]

Several case-control studies have demonstrated an association between high-risk HPV infection and the risk of HNSCC, independent of tobacco and alcohol use.[116–119] Moreover, HPV16 has been the most strongly associated HPV serotype with risk of HNC. A multicenter case-control study investigating the presence of HPV in oral and oropharyngeal cancers, compared 1670 cases with 1732 control subjects from nine countries and found that the presence of HPV16 markers conferred a significantly increased risk of HNC, and was correlated most strongly with oropharyngeal cancer (highest risk reported for E6 and E7 positivity: OR, 67.1; 95% CI, 12.9–348.2; compared with oral cavity cancer: OR, 4.3; 95% CI, 0.8–23.2).[118] However, an interplay between smoking and HPV-positive HNC exists, because national-level data indicate that 63.3% of HPV-positive oropharyngeal malignancies arose in ever-smokers compared with 36.7% among never-smokers (incidence 4.2 vs 2.3 per 100,000 person-years; relative risk, 1.81; 95% CI, 1.32–2.47).[120]

Betel Leaf and Area Nut

Historically, betel leaf and areca nut chewing has been a common socially accepted habit in South Asia, Southeast Asia, and Pacific Asia, and emigrated communities[121] in North America, Europe, and Africa in men and women and even in children, and is often retained in migrants from this area.[122,123] The prevalence of betel quid use is estimated to 10% to 20% of the world's population and 600 million chew areca nut.[124] To better qualify the risk associated with the use of each of these entities it is important to understand the correct terminology. Betel quid, otherwise known as pan or paan, is a term used to refer to a mixture of betel leaf, areca nut, aqueous calcium hydroxide paste (or slaked lime), and sometimes tobacco (referred to as gutka when containing tobacco).[125] Tobacco and/or areca nut act as the psychoactive component of betel quid. In fact, betel quid is the fourth most commonly used psychoactive substance after caffeine, alcohol, and nicotine.[122] Areca refers to a genus of palm trees that produce a fruit referred to as areca nut. The nut is consumed raw, or processed by sun-drying, baking, roasting, boiling, or fermenting. Betel quid chewing is associated with a characteristic reddish discoloration of the teeth and gingiva, which results from a chemical reaction that occurs as a result of mixing areca nut with slaked lime. Betel chewer's mucosa is a term that has been used to describe these characteristic changes, which include a brownish-red staining of the oral mucosa, irregularity of the mucosal surface, and desquamation of affected mucosa.[126] Betel chewer's mucosa is often found alongside leukoedema, leukoplakia, oral ulceration, and submucous fibrosis[127] and has the potential for malignant transformation. In fact, submucous fibrosis has been shown to convert to malignancies in 3% to 19%[127,128] and betel quid has been classified as a human carcinogen of the oral cavity, pharynx, and esophagus by the IARC.[125] In fact, use of betel quid with or without tobacco has been shown to confer a relative risk of oral cavity cancer greater than 50%, with the buccal mucosa, alveolar gingiva, and lip showing the highest risk of malignancy.[124]

Oral Hygiene

Avoidance of professional dental care, noncompliance to recommended dental care habits (eg, flossing and tooth brushing), missing dentition, and other markers of poor oral health have been repeatedly shown to be positively correlated and should be considered as an independent risk factor for increased risk of HNC, especially oral cancer.[129–132] An interesting and clinically relevant study by Chang and coworkers[133] performed a case control study comparing oral hygiene, as assessed through an interview, a questionnaire, and physical examination, in 317 HNC patients with 296 control subjects. They also administered a four-point standardized dental care habits and oral health score that consisted of (1) regular dental visits (yes/no), (2) tooth brushing (two or more times a day vs <2 times a day), (3) use of dental floss (yes/no), and (4) use of mouthwash (yes for alcohol-free vs no or use of alcohol-containing mouthwash). After adjusting for age and sex, they found that HNC was correlated with an absence of regular dental visits (OR, 2.86; 95% CI, 1.47–5.57), brushing less than two times a day (OR, 1.51; 95% CI, 1.02–2.23), absence of dental floss use (OR, 2.13; 95% CI, 1.47–3.09), frequent gum bleeding (OR, 3.15; 95% CI, 1.36–7.28), and more than 20 teeth absent (OR, 2.31; 95% CI, 1.05–5.07).[133] After further controlling their analysis for additional factors, such as education, alcohol consumption, and betel quid and cigarette use, no regular dental visits and brushing teeth less than twice a day were still significantly associated with HNC risk (respectively OR, 2.86, 95% CI, 1.47–5.57 and 1.51, 95% CI, 1.02–2.23). Moreover, for each point of increase in the dental care score, the risk of HNC increased by 60% (P = .0002) and increasing number of missing teeth also showed a direct statistically significant correlation for increased HNC cancer risk.

HEALTH ADVOCACY AND FUTURE OUTLOOK

HNC is an important entity and is one of the sixth most commonly diagnosed cancer worldwide.[134] Moreover, 66% of HNCs are diagnosed at advanced stages (III or IV). With the incidence of certain HNC types on the rise, the number of deaths is poised to increase from an estimated 300,000 to 595,000 deaths per year worldwide.[134,135] Moreover, HNC are amenable to screening and risk modification endeavors because many risk factors are modified by lifestyle modification measures, such as smoking cessation and alcohol use counseling. The goal of a screening program would identify the presence of carcinoma at an earlier stage and therefore improve outcomes, such as survival.[134] In fact, smoking cessation for 1 to 4 years significantly decreases the risk of HNC (OR, 0.7; 95% CI, 0.61–0.81) compared with current smoking and an even greater decrease in malignancy risk for 20 years or more smoking cessation (OR, 0.23; 95% CI, 0.18–0.31). Likewise, alcohol cessation reduces the risk of HNC to that of never-drinkers at 20 years or more of alcohol avoidance compared with current drinking (OR, 0.6; 95% CI, 0.40–0.89).[136]

In developed countries, where HPV-positive cancers of the oropharynx are on the rise, such measures as education and vaccination are key to improving the long-term outlook and overall elimination of the disease. Patients with HPV-positive cancers tend to be younger, with decreased alcohol and tobacco use, and are typically more affluent than those with HPV-negative disease. HPV-related cancer prevention is

accomplished by two methods: primary prevention, which consists of prevention of persistent HPV infections and resultant precancerous lesions; or secondary prevention, which consists of identification of precancerous disease, a treatable, or cancer at a curable stage.[137] Because no precancerous stage for HPV-positive oropharyngeal carcinoma is identified,[2] secondary prevention for HPV-related disease is accomplished only by early detection of carcinoma aided by patient education and by appropriate clinical suspicion from first-line health providers. Primary prevention relies on the use of the HPV vaccine, which has been shown to be effective at decreasing the prevalence of HPV infections and precancerous lesions in mucosal sites susceptible to malignancies.[138,139] There is no difference in HPV positivity in the oral cavity in eligible girls compared with boys of the same teenage group.[140] Moreover, in adulthood the overall prevalence of HPV positivity from mucosal swabs in males has been found to be 72.9%, and is much higher in adult men than in women regardless of age.[141] For this, and other reasons including equity and effectiveness of disease prevention, the Rome consensus conference concluded in 2013 that vaccination of 12-year-old boys should be included in vaccination policies.[141] The Centers for Disease Control and Prevention has also made recommendations that boys and girls receive the HPV vaccinations (can be started at age 9).[142] The HPV vaccine is highly efficient at reducing the prevalence of HPV infection,[143] and although vaccination rates for the first dose have been increasing in adolescents, there is still a disparity in vaccinations between genders (males 56% vs females 65%), and low completion rates (43%).[144] Measures to improve HPV vaccination success have been implemented, such as decreasing the recommended number of doses from three to two for youth younger than 15 years of age,[142] and availability of a nine-valent vaccination with extended coverage of less common but pathologically high-risk serotypes.[145]

REFERENCES

1. Gillison ML. Human papillomavirus-related diseases: oropharynx cancers and potential implications for adolescent HPV vaccination. J Adolesc Health 2008;43(4 Suppl):S52–60.
2. Lydiatt WM, Patel SG, O'Sullivan B, et al. Head and neck cancers-major changes in the American Joint Committee on Cancer eighth edition cancer staging manual. CA Cancer J Clin 2017;67(2):122–37.
3. Winn DM, Lee YC, Hashibe M, et al, INHANCE Consortium. The INHANCE consortium: toward a

better understanding of the causes and mechanisms of head and neck cancer. Oral Dis 2015; 21(6):685–93.

4. SEER cancer stat facts: oral cavity and pharynx cancer. Available at: https://seer.cancer.gov/statfacts/html/oralcav.html. Accessed December 17, 2017.

5. Siegel RL, Miller KD, Jemal A. Cancer statistics, 2017. CA Cancer J Clin 2017;67(1):7–30.

6. Howlader N, NA, Krapcho M, et al, editors. SEER cancer statistics review, 1975-2014. April 2017; based on November 2016 SEER data submission, posted to the SEER web site. 2017. Available at: https://seer.cancer.gov/csr/1975_2014/. Accessed December 18, 2017.

7. SEER cancer stat facts: laryngeal cancer. Available at: http://seer.cancer.gov/statfacts/html/laryn.html. Accessed December 17, 2017.

8. Hashibe M, Brennan P, Benhamou S, et al. Alcohol drinking in never users of tobacco, cigarette smoking in never drinkers, and the risk of head and neck cancer: pooled analysis in the International Head and Neck Cancer Epidemiology Consortium. J Natl Cancer Inst 2007;99(10):777–89.

9. Freedman ND, Schatzkin A, Leitzmann MF, et al. Alcohol and head and neck cancer risk in a prospective study. Br J Cancer 2007;96(9):1469–74.

10. Altieri A, Garavello W, Bosetti C, et al. Alcohol consumption and risk of laryngeal cancer. Oral Oncol 2005;41(10):956–65.

11. Talamini R, Bosetti C, La Vecchia C, et al. Combined effect of tobacco and alcohol on laryngeal cancer risk: a case-control study. Cancer Causes Control 2002;13(10):957–64.

12. Guzzo M, Locati LD, Prott FJ, et al. Major and minor salivary gland tumors. Crit Rev Oncol Hematol 2010;74(2):134–48.

13. Thom JJ, Moore EJ, Price DL, et al. The role of total parotidectomy for metastatic cutaneous squamous cell carcinoma and malignant melanoma. JAMA Otolaryngol Head Neck Surg 2014;140(6):548–54.

14. Spiro RH. Salivary neoplasms: overview of a 35-year experience with 2,807 patients. Head Neck Surg 1986;8(3):177–84.

15. Boukheris H, Curtis RE, Land CE, et al. Incidence of carcinoma of the major salivary glands according to the WHO classification, 1992 to 2006: a population-based study in the United States. Cancer Epidemiol Biomarkers Prev 2009;18(11):2899–906.

16. Yoo GH, Eisele DW, Askin FB, et al. Warthin's tumor: a 40-year experience at The Johns Hopkins Hospital. Laryngoscope 1994;104(7):799–803.

17. Land CE, Saku T, Hayashi Y, et al. Incidence of salivary gland tumors among atomic bomb survivors, 1950-1987. Evaluation of radiation-related risk. Radiat Res 1996;146(1):28–36.

18. Belsky JL, Tachikawa K, Cihak RW, et al. Salivary gland tumors in atomic bomb survivors, Hiroshima-Nagasaki, 1957 to 1970. JAMA 1972; 219(7):864–8.

19. Preston-Martin S, Thomas DC, White SC, et al. Prior exposure to medical and dental x-rays related to tumors of the parotid gland. J Natl Cancer Inst 1988;80(12):943–9.

20. Preston-Martin S, White SC. Brain and salivary gland tumors related to prior dental radiography: implications for current practice. J Am Dent Assoc 1990;120(2).151–8.

21. Modan B, Chetrit A, Alfandary E, et al. Increased risk of salivary gland tumors after low-dose irradiation. Laryngoscope 1998;108(7):1095–7.

22. Hoffman DA, McConahey WM, Fraumeni JF Jr, et al. Cancer incidence following treatment of hyperthyroidism. Int J Epidemiol 1982;11(3):218–24.

23. Saluja K, Butler RT, Pytynia KB, et al. Mucoepidermoid carcinoma post-radioactive iodine treatment of papillary thyroid carcinoma: unique presentation and putative etiologic association. Hum Pathol 2017;68:189–92.

24. Horn-Ross PL, Morrow M, Ljung BM. Menstrual and reproductive factors for salivary gland cancer risk in women. Epidemiology 1999;10(5):528–30.

25. Zheng W, Shu XO, Ji BT, et al. Diet and other risk factors for cancer of the salivary glands: a population-based case-control study. Int J Cancer 1996;67(2):194–8.

26. Dietz A, Barme B, Gewelke U, et al. The epidemiology of parotid tumors. A case control study. HNO 1993;41(2):83–90 [in German].

27. Turner JH, Reh DD. Incidence and survival in patients with sinonasal cancer: a historical analysis of population-based data. Head Neck 2012;34(6): 877–85.

28. Waldron J, Witterick I. Paranasal sinus cancer: caveats and controversies. World J Surg 2003;27(7): 849–55.

29. Voss R, Stenersen T, Roald Oppedal B, et al. Sinonasal cancer and exposure to softwood. Acta Otolaryngol 1985;99(1–2):172–8.

30. Innos K, Rahu M, Rahu K, et al. Wood dust exposure and cancer incidence: a retrospective cohort study of furniture workers in Estonia. Am J Ind Med 2000;37(5):501–11.

31. Gordon I, Boffetta P, Demers PA. A case study comparing a meta-analysis and a pooled analysis of studies of sinonasal cancer among wood workers. Epidemiology 1998;9(5):518–24.

32. Partanen T. Formaldehyde exposure and respiratory cancer: a meta-analysis of the epidemiologic evidence. Scand J Work Environ Health 1993; 19(1):8–15.

33. Luce D, Leclerc A, Begin D, et al. Sinonasal cancer and occupational exposures: a pooled analysis of 12 case-control studies. Cancer Causes Control 2002;13(2):147–57.

34. Olsen JH. Occupational risks of sinonasal cancer in Denmark. Br J Ind Med 1988;45(5):329–35.

35. Selden AI, Westberg HB, Axelson O. Cancer morbidity in workers at aluminum foundries and secondary aluminum smelters. Am J Ind Med 1997;32(5):467–77.

36. Karjalainen S, Kerttula R, Pukkala E. Cancer risk among workers at a copper/nickel smelter and nickel refinery in Finland. Int Arch Occup Environ Health 1992;63(8):547–51.

37. Slack R, Young C, Rushton L, British Occupational Cancer Burden Study Group. Occupational cancer in Britain. Nasopharynx and sinonasal cancers. Br J Cancer 2012;107(Suppl 1):S49–55.

38. 't Mannetje A, Kogevinas M, Luce D, et al. Sinonasal cancer, occupation, and tobacco smoking in European women and men. Am J Ind Med 1999;36(1):101–7.

39. Hayes RB, Kardaun JW, de Bruyn A. Tobacco use and sinonasal cancer: a case-control study. Br J Cancer 1987;56(6):843–6.

40. Thavaraj S. Human papillomavirus-associated neoplasms of the sinonasal tract and nasopharynx. Semin Diagn Pathol 2016;33(2):104–11.

41. Yu HX, Liu G. Malignant transformation of sinonasal inverted papilloma: a retrospective analysis of 32 cases. Oncol Lett 2014;8(6):2637–41.

42. Syrjanen K, Syrjanen S. Detection of human papillomavirus in sinonasal papillomas: systematic review and meta-analysis. Laryngoscope 2013; 123(1):181–92.

43. World Health Organization. WHO report on the global tobacco epidemic, 2013. 2013. Available at: http://apps.who.int/iris/bitstream/10665/85380/1/9789241505871_eng.pdf?ua=1. Accessed December 24, 2017.

44. IARC Working Group on the Evaluation of Carcinogenic Risks to Humans. Tobacco smoke and involuntary smoking. IARC Monogr Eval Carcinog Risks Hum 2004;83:1–1438.

45. Office of the Surgeon General (US), Office on Smoking and Health (US). The health consequences of smoking: a report of the surgeon general. Atlanta (GA): The Centers for Disease Control and Prevention (US); 2004.

46. World Health Organization, International Agency for Research on Cancer. [press release]. IARC strengthens its findings on several carcinogenic personal habits and household exposures. Lyons (France): WHO; 2009.

47. Preamble to the IARC monographs. 2006. Available at: http://monographs.iarc.fr/ENG/Preamble/current b6evalrationale0706.php. Accessed December 24, 2017.

48. International Agency for Research on Cancer. World cancer report. Lyons (France): IARC; 2014.

49. Oreggia F, De Stefani E, Correa P, et al. Risk factors for cancer of the tongue in Uruguay. Cancer 1991; 67(1):180–3.

50. IARC Working Group on the Evaluation of Carcinogenic Risks to Humans. Diesel and gasoline engine exhausts and some nitroarenes. IARC monographs on the evaluation of carcinogenic risks to humans. IARC Monogr Eval Carcinog Risks Hum 2014;105: 9–699.

51. De Stefani E, Boffetta P, Oreggia F, et al. Smoking patterns and cancer of the oral cavity and pharynx: a case-control study in Uruguay. Oral Oncol 1998; 34(5):340–6.

52. Franceschi S, Barra S, La Vecchia C, et al. Risk factors for cancer of the tongue and the mouth. A case-control study from northern Italy. Cancer 1992;70(9):2227–33.

53. Berthiller J, Straif K, Agudo A, et al. Low frequency of cigarette smoking and the risk of head and neck cancer in the INHANCE consortium pooled analysis. Int J Epidemiol 2016;45(3):835–45.

54. Wyss A, Hashibe M, Chuang SC, et al. Cigarette, cigar, and pipe smoking and the risk of head and neck cancers: pooled analysis in the International Head and Neck Cancer Epidemiology Consortium. Am J Epidemiol 2013;178(5):679–90.

55. IARC Working Group on the Evaluation of Carcinogenic Risks to Humans. Smokeless tobacco and some tobacco-specific N-nitrosamines. IARC Monogr Eval Carcinog Risks Hum 2007;89:1–592.

56. Phillips E, Wang TW, Husten CG, et al. Tobacco product use among adults: United States, 2015. MMWR Morb Mortal Wkly Rep 2017;66(44):1209–15.

57. Adriaens K, Van Gucht D, Declerck P, et al. Effectiveness of the electronic cigarette: an eight-week Flemish study with six-month follow-up on smoking reduction, craving and experienced benefits and complaints. Int J Environ Res Public Health 2014; 11(11):11220–48.

58. Hatsukami DK, Lemmonds C, Tomar SL. Smokeless tobacco use: harm reduction or induction approach? Prev Med 2004;38(3):309–17.

59. Stratton K, Shetty P, Wallace R, et al, editors. Clearing the smoke: assessing the science base for tobacco harm reduction. The National Academies Press: Washington, DC; 2001.

60. Cullen JW, Blot W, Henningfield J, et al. Health consequences of using smokeless tobacco: summary of the Advisory Committee's report to the Surgeon General. Public Health Rep 1986;101(4):355–73.

61. Hecht SS, Rivenson A, Braley J, et al. Induction of oral cavity tumors in F344 rats by tobacco-specific nitrosamines and snuff. Cancer Res 1986;46(8): 4162–6.

62. Rodu B, Cole P. Smokeless tobacco use and cancer of the upper respiratory tract. Oral Surg Oral Med Oral Pathol Oral Radiol Endod 2002;93(5):511–5.

63. Barraza LF, Weidenaar KE, Cook LT, et al. Regulations and policies regarding e-cigarettes. Cancer 2017;123(16):3007–14.

64. Vaporizers, E-Cigarettes, and other Electronic Nicotine Delivery Systems (ENDS). Available at: https://www.fda.gov/TobaccoProducts/Labeling/ProductsIngredientsComponents/ucm456610.htm. Accessed January 15, 2018.

65. Schoenborn CA, Gindi RM. Electronic cigarette use among adults. Hyattsville (MD): National Center for Health Statistics; 2015.

66. Miech RA, Johnston LD, O'Malley PM, et al. Monitoring the future national survey results on drug use, 1975-2016. Ann Arbor (MI): Institute for Social Research, The University of Michigan; 2017.

67. Pepper JK, Emery SL, Ribisl KM, et al. How risky is it to use e-cigarettes? Smokers' beliefs about their health risks from using novel and traditional tobacco products. J Behav Med 2015;38(2):318–26.

68. Franks AM, Hawes WA, McCain KR, et al. Electronic cigarette use, knowledge, and perceptions among health professional students. Curr Pharm Teach Learn 2017;9(6):1003–9.

69. Jamal A, Gentzke A, Hu SS, et al. Tobacco use among middle and high school students—United States, 2011-2016. MMWR Morb Mortal Wkly Rep 2017;66(23):597–603.

70. Yu V, Rahimy M, Korrapati A, et al. Electronic cigarettes induce DNA strand breaks and cell death independently of nicotine in cell lines. Oral Oncol 2016;52:58–65.

71. Holliday R, Kist R, Bauld L. E-cigarette vapour is not inert and exposure can lead to cell damage. Evid Based Dent 2016;17(1):2–3

72. Summary of Federal Rules for Tobacco Retailers. Available at: https://www.fda.gov/TobaccoProducts/GuidanceComplianceRegulatoryInformation/Retail/ucm205021.htm - ecig. Accessed December 24, 2017.

73. Hartmann-Boyce J, McRobbie H, Bullen C, et al. Electronic cigarettes for smoking cessation. Cochrane Database Syst Rev 2016;(9):CD010216.

74. Bullen C, Howe C, Laugesen M, et al. Electronic cigarettes for smoking cessation: a randomised controlled trial. Lancet 2013;382(9905):1629–37.

75. Caponnetto P, Campagna D, Cibella F, et al. Efficiency and safety of an eLectronic cigAreTte (ECLAT) as tobacco cigarettes substitute: a prospective 12-month randomized control design study. PLoS One 2013;8(6):e66317.

76. Primack BA, Shensa A, Sidani JE, et al. Initiation of traditional cigarette smoking after electronic cigarette use among tobacco-naïve U.S. young adults. Am J Med 2018;131(4):443.e1-9.

77. Schrot RJ, Hubbard JR. Cannabinoids: medical implications. Ann Med 2016;48(3):128–41.

78. NIDA. Marijuana. National Institute on Drug Abuse website. Available at: https://www.drugabuse.gov/drugs-abuse/marijuana. Accessed December 24, 2017.

79. Aldington S, Harwood M, Cox B, et al. Cannabis use and risk of lung cancer: a case-control study. Eur Respir J 2008;31(2):280–6.

80. Polen MR, Sidney S, Tekawa IS, et al. Health care use by frequent marijuana smokers who do not smoke tobacco. West J Med 1993;158(6):596–601.

81. Busch FW, Seid DA, Wei ET. Mutagenic activity of marihuana smoke condensates. Cancer Lett 1979;6(6):319–24.

82. Zhang ZF, Morgenstern H, Spitz MR, et al. Marijuana use and increased risk of squamous cell carcinoma of the head and neck. Cancer Epidemiol Biomarkers Prev 1999;8(12):1071–8.

83. Rosenblatt KA, Daling JR, Chen C, et al. Marijuana use and risk of oral squamous cell carcinoma. Cancer Res 2004;64(11):4049–54.

84. Llewellyn CD, Linklater K, Bell J, et al. An analysis of risk factors for oral cancer in young people: a case-control study. Oral Oncol 2004;40(3):304–13.

85. Hashibe M, Morgenstern H, Cui Y, et al. Marijuana use and the risk of lung and upper aerodigestive tract cancers: results of a population-based case-control study. Cancer Epidemiol Biomarkers Prev 2006;15(10):1829–34.

86. Aldington S, Harwood M, Cox B, et al. Cannabis use and cancer of the head and neck: case-control study. Otolaryngol Head Neck Surg 2008;138(3):374–80.

87. Llewellyn CD, Johnson NW, Warnakulasuriya KA. Risk factors for oral cancer in newly diagnosed patients aged 45 years and younger: a case-control study in Southern England. J Oral Pathol Med 2004;33(9):525–32.

88. Gillison ML, D'Souza G, Westra W, et al. Distinct risk factor profiles for human papillomavirus type 16-positive and human papillomavirus type 16-negative head and neck cancers. J Natl Cancer Inst 2008;100(6):407–20.

89. Committee on Substance Abuse, Committee on Adolescence, Committee on Substance Abuse Committee on Adolescence. The impact of marijuana policies on youth: clinical, research, and legal update. Pediatrics 2015;135(3):584–7.

90. Monte AA, Zane RD, Heard KJ. The implications of marijuana legalization in Colorado. JAMA 2015;313(3):241–2.

91. D'Souza DC, Ranganathan M. Medical marijuana: is the cart before the horse? JAMA 2015;313(24):2431–2.

92. Hall W, Degenhardt L. Adverse health effects of non-medical cannabis use. Lancet 2009;374(9698):1383–91.

93. Goldstein BY, Chang SC, Hashibe M, et al. Alcohol consumption and cancers of the oral cavity and pharynx from 1988 to 2009: an update. Eur J Cancer Prev 2010;19(6):431–65.

94. Boeing H, EPIC Working Group on Dietary Patterns. Alcohol and risk of cancer of the upper gastrointestinal tract: first analysis of the EPIC data. IARC Sci Publ 2002;156:151–4.

95. Alcohol drinking. IARC Working Group, Lyon, 13-20 October 1987. IARC Monogr Eval Carcinog Risks Hum 1988;44:1–378.

96. Koch WM, McQuone S. Clinical and molecular aspects of squamous cell carcinoma of the head and neck in the nonsmoker and nondrinker. Curr Opin Oncol 1997;9(3):257–61.

97. Blot WJ, McLaughlin JK, Winn DM, et al. Smoking and drinking in relation to oral and pharyngeal cancer. Cancer Res 1988;48(11):3282–7.

98. Schatzkin A, Subar AF, Thompson FE, et al. Design and serendipity in establishing a large cohort with wide dietary intake distributions: the National Institutes of Health-American Association of Retired Persons Diet and Health Study. Am J Epidemiol 2001;154(12):1119–25.

99. Burd EM. Human papillomavirus and cervical cancer. Clin Microbiol Rev 2003;16(1):1–17.

100. IARC Working Group on the Evaluation of Carcinogenic Risks to Humans. Human papillomaviruses. IARC Monogr Eval Carcinog Risks Hum 2007;90: 1–636.

101. Satterwhite CL, Torrone E, Meites E, et al. Sexually transmitted infections among US women and men: prevalence and incidence estimates, 2008. Sex Transm Dis 2013;40(3):187–93.

102. de Sanjose S, Diaz M, Castellsague X, et al. Worldwide prevalence and genotype distribution of cervical human papillomavirus DNA in women with normal cytology: a meta-analysis. Lancet Infect Dis 2007;7(7):453–9.

103. Hinchliffe SA, van Velzen D, Korporaal H, et al. Transience of cervical HPV infection in sexually active, young women with normal cervicovaginal cytology. Br J Cancer 1995;72(4):943–5.

104. Moscicki AB, Shiboski S, Broering J, et al. The natural history of human papillomavirus infection as measured by repeated DNA testing in adolescent and young women. J Pediatr 1998;132(2):277–84.

105. Flores ER, Allen-Hoffmann BL, Lee D, et al. Establishment of the human papillomavirus type 16 (HPV-16) life cycle in an immortalized human foreskin keratinocyte cell line. Virology 1999;262(2):344–54.

106. Gao G, Smith DI. Human papillomavirus and the development of different cancers. Cytogenet Genome Res 2016;150(3–4):185–93.

107. Munoz N, Castellsague X, de Gonzalez AB, et al. Chapter 1: HPV in the etiology of human cancer. Vaccine 2006;24(Suppl 3):S3/1-10.

108. Klussmann JP, Gultekin E, Weissenborn SJ, et al. Expression of p16 protein identifies a distinct entity of tonsillar carcinomas associated with human papillomavirus. Am J Pathol 2003;162(3):747–53.

109. Gillison ML, Koch WM, Capone RB, et al. Evidence for a causal association between human papillomavirus and a subset of head and neck cancers. J Natl Cancer Inst 2000;92(9):709–20.

110. El-Mofty SK. Human papillomavirus-related head and neck squamous cell carcinoma variants. Semin Diagn Pathol 2015;32(1):23–31.

111. Dahlstrom KR, Adler-Storthz K, Etzel CJ, et al. Human papillomavirus type 16 infection and squamous cell carcinoma of the head and neck in never-smokers: a matched pair analysis. Clin Cancer Res 2003;9(7):2620–6.

112. Stevens TM, Bishop JA. HPV-related carcinomas of the head and neck: morphologic features, variants, and practical considerations for the surgical pathologist. Virchows Arch 2017;471(2):295–307.

113. Carpén T, Sjöblom A, Lundberg M, et al. Presenting symptoms and clinical findings in HPV-positive and HPV-negative oropharyngeal cancer patients. Acta Otolaryngol 2018;138(5):513–8.

114. Westra WH. The morphologic profile of HPV-related head and neck squamous carcinoma: implications for diagnosis, prognosis, and clinical management. Head Neck Pathol 2012;6(Suppl 1):S48–54.

115. Jackson RS, Sinha P, Zenga J, et al. Transoral resection of human papillomavirus (HPV)-positive squamous cell carcinoma of the oropharynx: outcomes with and without adjuvant therapy. Ann Surg Oncol 2017;24(12):3494–501.

116. D'Souza G, Kreimer AR, Viscidi R, et al. Case-control study of human papillomavirus and oropharyngeal cancer. N Engl J Med 2007;356(19):1944–56.

117. Schwartz SM, Daling JR, Doody DR, et al. Oral cancer risk in relation to sexual history and evidence of human papillomavirus infection. J Natl Cancer Inst 1998;90(21):1626–36.

118. Herrero R, Castellsague X, Pawlita M, et al. Human papillomavirus and oral cancer: the International Agency for Research on Cancer multicenter study. J Natl Cancer Inst 2003;95(23):1772–83.

119. Smith EM, Ritchie JM, Summersgill KF, et al. Human papillomavirus in oral exfoliated cells and risk of head and neck cancer. J Natl Cancer Inst 2004;96(6):449–55.

120. Chaturvedi AK, D'Souza G, Gillison ML, et al. Burden of HPV-positive oropharynx cancers among ever and never smokers in the U.S. population. Oral Oncol 2016;60:61–7.

121. Shi LL, Bradford E, Depalo DE, et al. Betel quid use and oral cancer in a high-risk refugee community in the USA: the effectiveness of an awareness initiative. J Cancer Educ 2017. [Epub ahead of print].

122. Gupta PC, Ray CS. Epidemiology of betel quid usage. Ann Acad Med Singapore 2004;33(4 Suppl): 31–6.

123. Krais S, Klima M, Huppertz LM, et al. Betel nut chewing in Iron Age Vietnam? Detection of areca catechu alkaloids in dental enamel. J Psychoactive Drugs 2017;49(1):11–7.

124. Gupta PC, Warnakulasuriya S. Global epidemiology of areca nut usage. Addict Biol 2002;7(1): 77–83.

125. IARC Working Group on the Evaluation of Carcinogenic Risks to Humans. Betel-quid and areca-nut chewing and some areca-nut derived nitrosamines. IARC Monogr Eval Carcinog Risks Hum 2004;85:1–334.

126. Reichart PA, Phillipsen HP. Betel chewer's mucosa: a review. J Oral Pathol Med 1998;27(6):239–42.

127. Reichart PA, Mohr U, Srisuwan S, et al. Precancerous and other oral mucosal lesions related to chewing, smoking and drinking habits in Thailand. Community Dent Oral Epidemiol 1987;15(3):152–60.

128. Saravanan K, Kodanda Ram M, Ganesh R. Molecular biology of oral sub mucous fibrosis. J Cancer Res Ther 2013;9(2):179–80.

129. Franco EL, Kowalski LP, Oliveira BV, et al. Risk factors for oral cancer in Brazil: a case-control study. Int J Cancer 1989;43(6):992–1000.

130. Marshall JR, Graham S, Haughey BP, et al. Smoking, alcohol, dentition and diet in the epidemiology of oral cancer. Eur J Cancer B Oral Oncol 1992; 28B(1):9–15.

131. Rosenquist K, Wennerberg J, Schildt EB, et al. Oral status, oral infections and some lifestyle factors as risk factors for oral and oropharyngeal squamous cell carcinoma. A population-based case control study in Southern Sweden. Acta Otolaryngol 2005;125(12):1327–36.

132. Lissowska J, Pilarska A, Pilarski P, et al. Smoking, alcohol, diet, dentition and sexual practices in the epidemiology of oral cancer in Poland. Eur J Cancer Prev 2003;12(1):25–33.

133. Chang JS, Lo HI, Wong TY, et al. Investigating the association between oral hygiene and head and neck cancer. Oral Oncol 2013;49(10):1010–7.

134. Gogarty DS, Shuman A, O'Sullivan EM, et al. Conceiving a national head and neck cancer screening programme. J Laryngol Otol 2016; 130(1):8–14.

135. Mehanna H, Paleri V, West CM, et al. Head and neck cancer–Part 1: epidemiology, presentation, and prevention. BMJ 2010;341:c4684.

136. Marron M, Boffetta P, Zhang ZF, et al. Cessation of alcohol drinking, tobacco smoking and the reversal of head and neck cancer risk. Int J Epidemiol 2010; 39(1):182–96.

137. Kreimor AR. Prospects for prevention of HPV-driven oropharynx cancer. Oral Oncol 2014;50(6): 555–9.

138. Herrero R, Quint W, Hildesheim A, et al. Reduced prevalence of oral human papillomavirus (HPV) 4 years after bivalent HPV vaccination in a randomized clinical trial in Costa Rica. PLoS One 2013; 8(7):e68329.

139. Herrero R, Hildesheim A, Rodriguez AC, et al. Rationale and design of a community-based double-blind randomized clinical trial of an HPV 16 and 18 vaccine in Guanacaste, Costa Rica. Vaccine 2008;26(37):4795–808.

140. Durzynska J, Pacholska-Bogalska J, Kaczmarek M, et al. HPV genotypes in the oral cavity/oropharynx of children and adolescents: cross-sectional survey in Poland. Eur J Pediatr 2011;170(6):757–61.

141. Lenzi A, Mirone V, Gentile V, et al. Rome Consensus Conference: statement; human papilloma virus diseases in males. BMC Public Health 2013;13:117.

142. Clinician FAQs: CDC recommendations for HPV vaccine 2-dose schedule. Available at: https://www.cdc.gov/hpv/downloads/HCVG15-PTT-HPV-2Dose.pdf. Accessed December 25, 2017.

143. Markowitz LE, Hariri S, Lin C, et al. Reduction in human papillomavirus (HPV) prevalence among young women following HPV vaccine introduction in the United States, National Health and Nutrition Examination Surveys, 2003-2010. J Infect Dis 2013;208(3):385–93.

144. HPV vaccination coverage data. Available at: https://www.cdc.gov/hpv/hcp/vacc-coverage.html. Accessed December 25, 2017.

145. HPV vaccine information for clinicians. Available at: https://www.cdc.gov/hpv/hcp/need-to-know.pdf. Accessed December 25, 2017.

Framework for Speech–Language Pathology Services in Patients with Oral Cavity and Oropharyngeal Cancers

Loni C. Arrese, PhD[a], Katherine A. Hutcheson, PhD[b],*

KEYWORDS

- Speech–language pathology • Dysphagia • Dysarthria • Functional outcomes • Rehabilitation

KEY POINTS

- Speech and swallowing impairments take many forms in this population and are driven by tumor burden and location, treatment modality, comorbidities, and age.
- Baseline functional assessment with speech–language pathology is best practice for most patients diagnosed with oral cavity or oropharyngeal cancers.
- Postoperative rehabilitation needs vary greatly by procedure and patient; early initiation of postoperative rehabilitation is advocated.
- Radiotherapy generally has greater impact on swallowing over speech function in this population.
- Proactive swallowing therapy models are considered best practice to maximize pharyngeal activity through the duration of radiotherapy.

INTRODUCTION

This article provides a framework for speech–language pathology services in the assessment and treatment of patients with oral cavity and oropharynx cancers. For purposes of this article, we maintain the assumptions that (1) oral cavity cancers are primarily treated surgically as a single modality when early stage and typically require adjuvant radiotherapy (RT) or chemoradiation (CRT) for advanced stages of disease and that (2) oropharyngeal cancers are largely treated without surgery and often require multimodality treatment with shifting trends toward primary transoral resection in patients with low to intermediate risk disease.

NATURE OF THE PROBLEM

The complexity of the head and neck region involves an abundance of neurovascular structures responsible for breathing, speaking, and eating. Locoregional treatment modalities aim to eradicate head and neck tumors while intending to preserve these essential functions. However, treatment modalities for head and neck cancer (HNC), which include surgery, RT, and CRT, can impact both the anatomy as well as the tissue characteristics and neural inputs of the structures and muscles involved in speech and swallowing. Thus, speech and swallowing problems are among the most challenging functional deficits to rehabilitate after oncologic treatment for HNC.

Disclosure: The authors have nothing to disclose.
[a] Department of Otolaryngology - Head and Neck Surgery, Ohio State University, 320 West 10th Avenue, Columbus, OH 43210, USA; [b] Department of Head and Neck Surgery, The University of Texas MD Anderson Cancer Center, Houston, TX 77030, USA
* Corresponding author. Department of Head and Neck Surgery, The University of Texas MD Anderson Cancer Center, PO Box 301402, Unit 1445, Houston, TX 77230-1402.
E-mail address: karnold@mdanderson.org

Oral Maxillofacial Surg Clin N Am 30 (2018) 397–410
https://doi.org/10.1016/j.coms.2018.07.001
1042-3699/18/© 2018 Elsevier Inc. All rights reserved.

Much of the recent increase in prevalence of HNC is attributed to the growing epidemic of a virally mediated form of disease associated with the human papillomavirus (HPV).[1] Persistent HPV infection can alter immune function and cause genetic damage, which may progress to squamous cell carcinoma arising from the epithelial mucosa of the upper aerodigestive tract most typically in the oropharynx. This epidemiologic shift is impacting individuals (males > females; 3:1) primarily in their 40s and 50s who have no significant history of tobacco and/or alcohol use.[2] Fortunately, improved therapeutic response and increased survival are associated with HPV-related disease (HPV+).[3,4] However, outside of an investigational setting, treatment regimens and dosing presently remain equivalent to standards derived for populations with tobacco related HNC. Thus, clinicians currently face a growing population of young and otherwise healthy cancer survivors who are challenged by sometimes devastating, often long-term, consequences of HNC treatment, chief among these issues speech and swallowing deficits.

DYSPHAGIA

The incidence of dysphagia at time of HNC diagnosis is reported as high as 40%[5] and is often a direct consequence of tumor invasion into the swallowing musculature in patients with locally advanced tumors (baseline dysphagia is rare in patients with early stage disease). After diagnosis, dysphagia severity is then typically exacerbated, if present at diagnosis, or originated by oncologic treatment. Pretreatment dysphagia severity has been shown to correlate with disease stage,[6–8] whereas the severity of posttreatment dysphagia is directly related to the site of lesion, presence of neck metastasis, and the cancer treatment modality. Multimodality therapies are common practice for treatment of HNC, with approximately 80% of all patients with HNC receiving RT during the course of treatment for their disease.[9,10]

Dysphagia after RT is characterized by a decreased range of motion of the laryngopharyngeal structures involved in swallowing. RT targets rapidly dividing cancer cells while attempting to spare slower dividing somatic cells. Acute and late effects of radiation on normal tissues depend on many factors, such as the RT field, dose per fraction, number of fractions (including fractions per day), interfraction interval, total dose, and the duration over which the dose is delivered. Muscles critical to swallowing often overlap RT targets or are in close proximity such that bystander dose is unavoidable. Conformal methods of delivery, such as intensity-modulated radiation therapy and volumetric arch therapy, among others, are now the standard of care for delivery of RT to patients with HNC. This strategy allows for the delivery of a therapeutic dose to the tumor while protecting, as much as possible, the nearby dose-limiting structures, such as the orbital regions, eyes, parotid glands, and the dysphagia-aspiration related structures (ie, pharyngeal constrictors, larynx, and submental muscles).[11–14] Despite sparing of these dose-limiting structures, a low-dose "bath" of radiation to normal muscles occurs, delivering a low dose to various structures including nerves, ligaments, tendons, bones, as well as the vascular system within the radiation field.[13] As such, even with modern RT techniques, meaningful numbers of patients develop radiation-associated dysphagia (RAD) as a long-term consequence of this therapy. In oropharyngeal cancers, the severity of dysphagia is reported to impact quality of life[15] and decisional regret[16] about cancer treatment with larger effect sizes than other toxicities.

After CRT, it is estimated that 39% to 64% of patients have chronic swallowing deficits.[17–19] Dysphagia presents as the primary functional concern for this patient population,[20] drives perception of quality of life after CRT and significantly predicts for pneumonia during long-term survivorship.[21] Specific to patients with primary tumors of the oropharynx, it is estimated that 7% to 31% develop chronic aspiration,[17,22] 11% develop aspiration pneumonia,[21] and 4% are chronically dependent on a feeding tube after CRT.[23] The high prevalence of dysphagia within this patient population further contributes to significant medical, psychosocial, and nutritional sequelae.

Functional outcomes after surgical resection for HNC vary significantly. However, surgical resection, with or without microvascular reconstruction, may yield more predictable functional outcomes specific to tumor size (clinical T stage) and location.[24] Advanced tumors (ie, T3-T4), requiring larger resection often result in worse postoperative function owing to the anatomic and neurophysiologic consequences of surgery.[25] Further, location of the surgical bed within the aerodigestive track directly relates to functional outcomes. In general, within the oral cavity and oropharynx, oral phase impairments are dominant after oral tongue and floor of the mouth resection, whereas pharyngeal phase impairments, including aspiration, are more prevalent succeeding base of tongue resection.[25]

SPEECH

Deficits in speech intelligibility for oral and oropharynx patients with cancer are often a result of (1) direct surgical excision of the structures responsible for articulation and resonance and/or (2) resultant from neuromuscular effects of RT such as fibrosis or cranial neuropathies. A systematic review of the literature suggests that surgical resection of oral or oropharyngeal cancer often results in aberrant, although intelligible speech production ranging from 92% to 98% intelligibility at the sentence level.[26] Speech outcomes primarily depend on the structure and function of both the soft palate for resonance and the oral tongue for articulation.[26,27] Lingual mobility and strength are associated with speech intelligibility after partial or hemiglossectomy that preserves greater than 50% of the native tongue, with increased mobility being associated with better outcomes.[26,28] After subtotal and total glossectomy, speech outcomes are highly variable.[26] However, with the use of microvascular free flap reconstruction, functional speech outcomes can be achieved and correlate with the bulk and contour of the reconstructed tongue.[29,30] In cases of maxillary resection (maxillectomy), the resultant hypernasality often affects articulation and speech intelligibility. Although intelligible speech production is most often achieved after surgical reconstruction or after prosthetic obturation to fill the oronasal defect,[31] patient-reported functional outcomes remain lower when compared with nontumor (not reconstructed or obturated) controls.[32]

Variability exists within the literature regarding speech outcomes after organ-sparing therapies.[26] However, radiation delivery to the aerodigestive and vocal tract can elicit tissue-related changes resulting in decreased range of motion of the articulators. Consequently, voice production and speech intelligibility may be impacted. Reduced speech intelligibility and impaired articulation are highly associated with reduced quality of life[33] and can be attributed to scarring, edema, and fibrosis of structures within the oral cavity or oropharynx.[34] Further, voice disturbances resulting from toxicities of RT including xerostomia and dryness of the laryngeal mucosa may impact functional status and quality of life in patients with HNC.[35]

THERAPEUTIC OPTIONS
Baseline Functional Assessment

Owing to the significant impact of cancer treatment on functional outcomes, including speech, swallowing, and quality of life, oncology providers increasingly recognize the importance of proactive speech–language pathology services.[6,36] Many high-volume HNC programs consider it best practice to include instrumental baseline assessment of swallowing function via videofluoroscopy or flexible endoscopic evaluation of swallowing in their multidisciplinary approach to patient and symptom management for patients at risk of posttreatment pharyngeal dysphagia. Baseline clinical speech testing and counseling are advised for patients planned for treatment expected to impact, even temporarily, articulation and/or resonance. Appropriate assessment in conjunction with timely, proactive intervention serves to reduce the severity or risk of adverse effects of cancer treatments. Additionally, baseline assessments can expose subclinical swallowing deficits related to impaired bolus efficiency and/or airway protection and allow for individualized swallowing-related treatment recommendations to optimize oral intake, establish appropriate patient-centered goals, and set realistic expectations for functional changes throughout cancer treatment (**Fig. 1**).

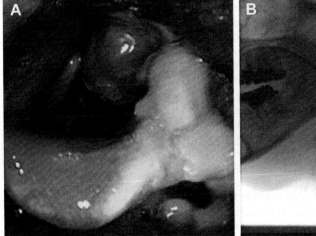
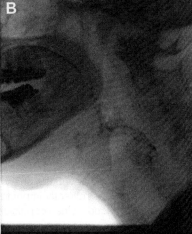

Fig. 1. Baseline assessment. (*A*) Endoscopic view of left sided supraglottic mass. (*B*) Radiographic view of mass effect yielding bolus efficiency (residue) and airway safety (aspiration) impairments.

Rehabilitation Considerations After Surgical Treatment (Oral Cavity Cancers)

Surgical resection of primary oral cavity tumors may alter an individual's cosmetic appearance, quality of life, and functionality, including the ability to talk, smell, chew, and/or swallow.[37–41] In general, postoperative functional outcomes are fairly predictable based on the location and size of the required resection (T stage), surgical approach (transoral vs conventional techniques), closure technique (primary closure vs reconstruction, including microvascular flap), and management of neck disease. Results from the baseline swallowing assessment combined with the operative documentation create a strong framework for dysphagia clinicians to establish appropriate dysphagia management. It is important to note that adjuvant RT or CRT is often required 4 to 6 weeks after definitive oral resection for advanced stages of disease. Adjuvant therapy exacerbates the postoperative side effects, particularly with regard to pharyngeal swallow function, and a critical goal is to prioritize as much swallowing progress as possible before adjuvant RT begins.

In the immediate postoperative phase, edema is common and can significantly impact the biomechanical coordination of essential structures in the oral cavity and aerodigestive tract for respiration and swallowing. The bulk of postoperative swelling often resolves within a few weeks, allowing for more intensive speech and swallowing rehabilitation.[24] Lymphedema, however, may begin to set in as early as 4 to 6 weeks after therapy, for which complete decongestive therapy is the standard.[42] The severity of lymphedema is significantly correlated with symptoms of dysphagia and speech impairment,[43] further motivating integration of lymphedema therapy into comprehensive rehabilitation.

Salient features of oral stage dysphagia after oral cavity resection are primarily characterized by impaired bolus acceptance or containment (eg, decreased mouth opening or poor labial function), prolonged bolus manipulation and transit times (eg, mastication, bolus collection), and impaired bolus clearance (eg, oral propulsion). These oral stage deficits typically warrant labial and lingual range of motion, agility, and strengthening exercise paradigms. Long-term airway safety compromise is less common after oral cavity surgery (particularly for low-volume tumors) than oropharyngeal surgery. However, the pharyngeal phase of swallow may be indirectly impacted by premature spillage, reduced bolus propulsion, and more directly impacted hyolaryngeal complex instability resulting in reduced laryngeal vestibule closure and impaired cricopharyngeal opening.

Surgical resection, specifically within the oral cavity, impacts speech intelligibility by way of articulation and resonance. Motor speech assessments by way of standardized articulation batteries (eg, the Fisher-Logemann Test of Articulation) are useful to determine rehabilitative targets for improved speech intelligibility. Speech rehabilitation relies heavily on compensatory techniques aimed to exaggerate movements of the remaining structures to improve articulatory contacts. Glossectomy-specific compensatory phonetic strategies pioneered by the work of Skelly and colleagues[44,45] in the 1970s remain useful in contemporary practice.[46] Assessment and response to early treatment may further assist with shaping and overall design of a palatal augmentation prostheses when warranted (**Table 1**).

Impact of Oral Prosthetic Devices on Speech and Swallowing

Oral prosthetic devices designed by a maxillofacial prosthodontist are intended to improve speech and swallowing outcomes in patients with (1) altered oral anatomy resulting from surgery or (2) impaired physiologic function resulting from surgery and/or CRT. Various types of oral and pharyngeal prosthetics serve to improve speech intelligibility and facilitate the oral phases of swallowing by way of improved chewing, bolus containment and formation, decreasing tongue to palate distance, and pharyngeal functions by improving velopharyngeal seal and increasing propulsive pressure on the bolus. Common prosthetic devices for patients with HNC include dentures, palatal-lowering devices (ie, palatal augmentation prostheses), palatal prosthesis with obturator (**Fig. 2**), and mandibular and lingual prosthetics. Collaboration between the prosthodontist and speech–language pathologist can ensure best speech and swallow-related functional outcomes.

With prosthetic rehabilitation, the speech–language pathologist assesses function before, during, and after the fitting of a prosthesis to guide contours. In addition to subjective measurements of speech intelligibility and swallowing function, instrumental examinations, particularly videofluoroscopy (for observation of oral contacts and efficiency) and endoscopy (for dynamic examination of velopharyngeal function) are used to assess the functionality of a prosthetic. Further, pressure measurements using the Iowa Oral Performance Instrument can determine the appropriate size and location of prosthetic bulk, particularly for palatal augmentation prostheses, to optimize speech and swallowing tasks. The impact of these prosthetic devices on speech and swallowing function is outlined herein.

Table 1
Potential impairments based on location of surgical resection

Surgical Location	Potential Impairment
Lip resection	Impaired approximation of orbicularis oris Oral containment difficulties; drooling Altered oral sphincter Distorted labial sound production
Floor of mouth resection	Loss of glossoalveolar sulcus Tethering of the anterior tongue → reduced lingual ROM Loss of dentition impacting masticating Impaired hyolaryngeal excursion Distorted velar and alveolar sound production
Tongue Resection	Impaired bolus preparation and transport Impaired driving force on the bolus Reduced lingual ROM → bolus pooling; impaired clearance through the oral cavity Impaired articulation
Mandibulectomy	Altered oral containment (if anterior) Loss of dentition Reduced chewing force
Hard palate resection	Loss of oronasal separation resulting in nasal regurgitation and resonance disturbance (hypernasality)
Soft palate resection	Velopharyngeal insufficiency resulting in nasal regurgitation and resonance disturbance (hypernasality) Loss of proximal seal for pharyngeal pressure propagation
Tonsil	Altered lateral pharyngeal wall movement Possible extension to soft palate with associated VPI concerns

Abbreviation: ROM, range of motion; VPI, velopharyngeal insufficiency.

- *Dentures*: Assist with bolus manipulation (mastication); improve quality of life; and provide articulatory contacts for improved speech intelligibility.[47]
- *Palatal-lowering prosthesis*: Reshapes the contour of the oral cavity; lowers the palatal vault to improve anatomic contacts for improved swallowing and speech production (ie, tongue to palate contact pressures).[48]
- *Obturators*: Diminishes difficulties related to mastication and swallowing[49]; improves speech intelligibility[26,50]; reduces the distance between the soft palate and the posterior tongue; lifts the soft palate to foster contact with the posterior and lateral pharyngeal walls; closes the port between the nasopharynx and oropharynx thus reducing nasal regurgitation during swallowing and restoring intrabolus pressure required for adequate bolus clearance.
- *Mandibular and lingual prosthetics*: Decreases the size of the oral cavity; contours the oral cavity for management of secretion; provides a framework for contact with the surrounding structures during speech and swallowing tasks; improves swallowing and speech intelligibility.[51–53]

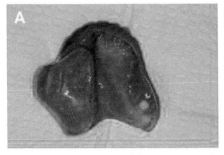
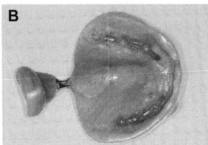

Fig. 2. Obturators. (*A*) Obturator to fill/reconstruct a hard palate defect. (*B*) Obturator to fill/reconstruct a soft palate defect or deficit.

Rehabilitation Considerations After Nonsurgical Treatment (Oropharyngeal Cancers)

Treatment for many sites of HNC, specifically within the oropharynx, has shifted over the past decades to focus on organ-sparing therapies using definitive radiation therapy with or without chemotherapy. Although conformal RT techniques have been proven effective to reduce xerostomia without a decrease in overall survival,[54,55] both acute and long-term adverse effects persist and particularly impact swallowing function and quality of life.[56,57] Acute side effects of radiation therapy include radiation dermatitis, pain, loss of energy, mucositis, soft tissue edema, weight loss, mucus, xerostomia, impaired taste, voice changes, muscle fibrosis, trismus, and dysphagia.[56]

In the acute phase of injury, structures within the radiation field become edematous. As vascular changes progress, there is a loss of muscle fibers, decrease in fiber size, necrosis, and stiffening of muscles (ie, fibrosis). These changes adversely impact the neuromuscular structures involved in swallowing,[58–60] resulting in RAD.[61] Further progression of the neuromuscular insult can result in persistent dysphagia or even late RAD, which can first present or progress substantially decades after RT. Late RAD is typically observed after the delayed onset of mononeuropathies or polyneuropathies of the lower cranial nerves, resulting in profound impairment.[61,62]

The framework for proactive speech–language pathology services in patients receiving definitive RT to the head and neck region (**Fig. 3**A) is recognized as best practice. It should be noted that swallowing rehabilitation (and prehabilitation) models are more mature in this area compared with other HNC populations. This section provides a basis for the proactive management of RAD as well as considerations for reactive rehabilitation of persistent and late RAD (**Fig. 3**B).

Speech–language pathology management of radiation or CRT patients can be divided into 3 timeframes: (1) baseline assessment and initiation

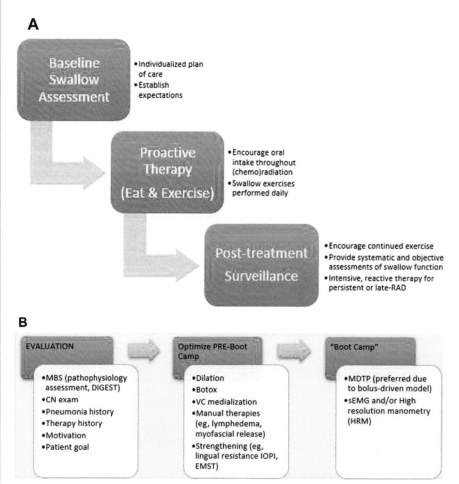

A

Baseline Swallow Assessment
- Individualized plan of care
- Establish expectations

Proactive Therapy (Eat & Exercise)
- Encourage oral intake throughout (chemo)radiation
- Swallow exercises performed daily

Post-treatment Surveillance
- Encourage continued exercise
- Provide systematic and objective assessments of swallow function
- Intensive, reactive therapy for persistent or late-RAD

B

EVALUATION
- MBS (pathophysiology assessment, DIGEST)
- CN exam
- Pneumonia history
- Therapy history
- Motivation
- Patient goal

Optimize PRE-Boot Camp
- Dilation
- Botox
- VC medialization
- Manual therapies (eg, lymphedema, myofascial release)
- Strengthening (eg, lingual resistance IOPI, EMST)

"Boot Camp"
- MDTP (preferred due to bolus-driven model)
- sEMG and/or High resolution manometry (HRM)

Fig. 3. (A) Framework for speech–language pathology services during radiotherapy or chemoradiotherapy. (B) Framework for boot camp swallowing therapy for persistent or late radiation-associated dysphagia (RAD). CN, cranial nerves; EMST, expiratory muscle stregnth training; IOPI, iowa oral performance instrument; MBS, modified barium swallow study; MDTP, mcNeill dysphagia therapy program; sEMG, surface electromyography; VC, vocal cord.

of proactive intervention, (2) early, intensive reactive therapy in response to persistent posttreatment RAD, and (3) surveillance, which may expose the onset of late RAD.

Proactive intervention

The literature examining the impact of proactive swallowing-related intervention is composed of retrospective, observational, and randomized clinical trials (**Table 2**).[63–70] It is important to note that data collection time points, outcome measures, swallowing interventions, and comparison groups (control group vs comparison to the literature) vary significantly between these studies yielding inconclusive results of a recent Cochrane review.[71]

In single studies, however, proactive swallowing exercise interventions are associated with superior long-term functional outcomes and, in many institutions, are currently recommended for patients with HNC receiving RT to bilateral neck fields in excess of 60 Gy in effort to reduce severity of chronic dysphagia by avoiding prolonged disuse of swallowing musculature during or after RT or CRT.

Acute dysphagia during and immediately after a course of CRT is typically considered to reflect the effects of oral mucositis, pain, edema, and possibly disuse atrophy. Mucositis results from the shedding of the outer epithelium cells at a rate that exceeds their replacement. Unfortunately, the incidence of mucositis resulting from

Table 2
Summary of studies examining efficacy of proactive swallowing exercise interventions for patients receiving RT or CRT for HNC

Author	Outcome Measures	Timing of Intervention	Results for the Exercise or Adherent Group
Kulbersh et al,[63] 2006	MD Anderson Dysphagia Inventory	2 wk before treatment	Improved QOL measures: physical, emotional, global No improved QOL in the functional domain
Carroll et al,[64] 2008	VFSS G-tube status	2 wk before treatment vs after treatment	Significant differences in epiglottic inversion and tongue position during swallow No difference in PEG removal
Kotz et al,[65] 2012	FOIS Performance Status Scale -H&N	At the start of treatment	Improved oral intake at time points 3 and 6 mo after treatment
Van der Molen et al,[66] 2011	VFSS Maximum mandibular opening Body mass index FOIS G-tube dependency Pain scale Study-specific questionnaire	2 wk before treatment	Demonstrated good feasibility of performing proactive swallowing exercises Reduced G-tube dependency
Carnaby-Mann et al,[67] 2012	Muscle size and composition Swallowing ability Dietary intake Chemosensory function Salivation Nutritional status Occurrence of dysphagia-related complications	At the start of treatment	Superior muscle composition on MRI and functional swallowing ability per MASA
Duarte et al,[68] 2013	Nutritional intake (chewable; puree; liquid; G-tube) Exercise adherence	2 wk before treatment	Majority taking regular "chewable" diet at 1 mo after treatment
Hutcheson et al,[69] 2013	Nutritional intake G-tube dependency Exercise adherence	Before treatment	Improved maintenance of regular diet in long-term survivorship and shorter G-tube dependency
Virani et al,[70] 2015	FOIS G-tube dependency	At the start of treatment	Reduced G-tube dependency

Abbreviations: CRT, chemoradiation; FIOS, Functional Oral Intake Scale; HNC, head and neck cancer; H&N, head and neck; QOL, quality of life; ROM, range of motion; RT, radiation therapy; VFSS, videofluoroscopy.

concurrent CRT for HNC is close to 100%, but the volume of tissue affected is contingent fully on the RT fields.[72,73] Mucositis symptoms include severe pain with swallowing (odynophagia) and salivary changes, often causing patients to expectorate their oral secretions and reduce their oral intake. It is theorized that diminished frequency of swallowing in response to acute toxicities negatively impacts the muscles of the aerodigestive tract by way of disuse atrophy.[69]

Hutcheson and colleagues[69] published that increased swallowing activity during RT (via maintenance of oral intake and swallowing exercise) is associated with higher probability of eating a regular oral diet in long-term survivorship after nonsurgical treatment for HNC. With multivariate analysis, these investigators further concluded that patients who either eat or performed swallowing exercises had superior functional status as compared with those who did neither, and patients who did both (eat and exercise) had the highest rate of return to a regular diet and the shortest duration of feeding tube dependence. Accordingly, speech–language pathology services during this acute phase of symptom management focus primarily on proactive swallowing therapy to (1) avoid intervals of immobilization and nil per os and (2) encourage performance of physiologically guided exercises designed to maximize use of the swallowing musculature.

Radiation- or CRT-induced dysphagia primarily depends on tumor size and the presence or absence of metastatic neck disease. These oncologic features greatly impact the radiation field and dose required for definitive treatment. Impaired base of tongue retraction, reduced hyolaryngeal elevation, and impaired contraction of the pharyngeal constrictors have been identified as the salient features of dysphagia after RT for HNC.[74] Thus, swallowing exercises specific to maintaining the range of motion and muscle mass of these structures are targeted throughout the continuum of dysphagia therapy.

Persistent radiation-associated dysphagia
Although most patients recover a functional level of swallowing ability and may attenuate their expectations to their posttreatment level of function (the "new normal"), approximately 35% to 40% experience persistent moderate to severe RAD in the absence of remaining disease.[75] Persistent dysphagia is a challenging problem that does not respond measurably to traditional low frequency, short durations of therapy (often carried out at home by the patient), but instead requires intensive daily therapy often using biofeedback,[76] bolus-driven therapy,[77,78] and/or device-driven therapy[79] paradigms to progressively challenge the

swallowing system. This aggressive approach to swallow recovery has been coined "boot camp" by MD Anderson using an algorithm to tailor published progressive therapy paradigms for dysphagia to meet the needs of the HNC survivor.[76–79]

The boot camp model simply arranges the available options (eg, biofeedback, bolus driven, and/or device driven) to systematically offer more intensive swallowing therapies when needed for persistent or late RAD. Boot camp swallowing therapy is thus a model to deliver intensive, clinician-directed swallowing therapy. In daily functional therapy, typically over 2 to 3 weeks, boot camp challenges the patient by mass practice of functional swallowing tasks with progressive loading. Progressive resistance is achieved using increasing bolus viscosity and size or both (per principals of the McNeill Dysphagia Therapy Program) and/or via biofeedback through surface electrical myography.[76–78] Before beginning functional boot camp therapy with the McNeill Dysphagia Therapy Program or biofeedback, any and all methods recommended to optimize the swallowing system should take place. These efforts might include medical/surgical procedures (eg, dilation or injection of botulinum toxin in the pharyngoesophageal segment), manual therapies, and/or a strengthening regimen for oral or laryngopharyngeal musculature. After optimization, in general, a bolus-driven functional therapy is preferred for boot camp (eg, McNeill Dysphagia Therapy Program) based on case-control data that suggest superior functional gains with bolus-driven rather than biofeedback-driven therapy[77] (see **Fig. 3**B).

Surveillance
Owing to discrepancy between patient perception and swallow pathophysiology,[80,81] a systematic approach of dysphagia surveillance that includes instrumental assessment is warranted for this patient population. This timing often mimics the National Comprehensive Cancer Network clinical practice guidelines for tumor surveillance.

The most likely late effect of treatment that merits speech pathology services is late RAD. Late RAD is a rare (likely <10% incidence) condition, commonly precipitated by delayed onset of treatment associated cranial neuropathies that have been published to occur with extreme latency in oropharyngeal cancer survivors (median onset, 7–9 years).[61,62,82] Case series suggest profoundly altered swallow physiology with late RAD and silent aspiration (poorly detected in clinic) is almost universally present when affected survivors are tested with videofluoroscopy or endoscopy (**Fig. 4**). This observation, coupled with a high probability of aspiration pneumonia in this

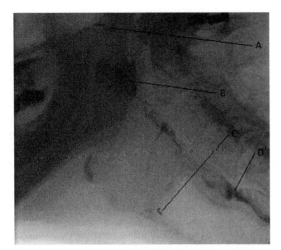

Fig. 4. Radiographic evidence of radiation-associated dysphagia (RAD). (A) Nasopharyngeal regurgitation. (B) Impaired base of tongue to posterior pharyngeal wall contact. (C) Silent aspiration. (D) Stricture.

population (>65%), suggests an impetus to refer long-term survivors with new or progressive dysphagia symptoms, clinical evidence of lower cranial neuropathy, and/or aspiration pneumonia for instrumental assessment (fluoroscopy or endoscopy) of swallowing with a speech pathologist.

COMPLICATIONS AND CONSIDERATIONS

Swallowing function and speech intelligibility are critical aspects of daily functioning. As such, temporary and especially chronic speech and swallowing dysfunction can have a profound impact on quality of life. HNC-induced dysphagia is not only a significant contributor to reduced quality of life, but it is also associated with major health and financial implications. These include enteral feeding dependency, hospitalizations, economic burden, and mortality. In this section, these associated ramifications of HNC-induced dysphagia are discussed.

Quality of Life

Speech and swallowing function drives quality of life in treated patients with HNC. Therefore, tracking and addressing a patient's perception of their functional status and quality of life is a critical aspect of patient-centered care. Patient perception often drives medical decision making and adherence to diet and exercise recommendations; thus, it is an essential aspect of a clinician's assessment and treatment planning. Patient-reported outcome questionnaires represent a standardized method to identify domain specific patient concerns and aid in the establishment of patient-centered goals. Detailed explanations of

the most common patient-reported outcomes are beyond the scope of this article; however, they are listed for reference in **Table 3**.[83–91]

Health and Financial Implications of Dysphagia

Malnutrition, defined as 5% to 10% unintentional weight loss within 1 to 6 months and a body mass index of 18.5 to 20 kg/m^2, is present in 3% to 52% of patients with HNC at the time of diagnosis and increases to 44% to 88% during CRT.[92] Treatment-related toxicities (eg, taste changes, xerostomia, and dysphagia) often further exacerbate nutritional status during treatment and into survivorship. Further, malnutrition leads to reduced quality of life[93] and has been linked to increased frequency and severity of RT-induced late toxicities,[94] including mortality.[95]

Regardless of treatment modality, alternative means of nutrition are often a necessity (at least temporarily) in the setting of significant malnutrition, dysphagia, and/or odynophagia. In the early stages of treatment, approximately 50% of patients with cancer receiving CRT require a feeding tube owing to pain, lack of appetite, and/or dysphagia.[96] Enteral feeding not only results in a reduced quality of life, but it is also yields a significant cost consequence, including hospital stay. Callahan and colleagues[97] conservatively estimated the total annual cost of percutaneous endoscopic gastrostomy (PEG) placement and tube feeding to be as much as $31,832. However, many patients have a shorter course of PEG tube dependency. Additionally, although enteral feeding is a means to provide adequate nutrition,

Table 3	
Patient-reported outcome questionnaires	
Perceived Swallowing	**MD Anderson Dysphagia Inventory (MDADI)**[83]
Impairment	The Eating Assessment Tool (EAT-10)[84]
Reported oral intake	The Performance Status Scale – Head and Neck (PSS-HN)[85] The Functional Oral Intake Scale (FOIS)[86]
Speech and voice	The Voice Handicap Index (VHI)[87] Speech Handicap Index (SHI)[88]
Dry mouth	Xerostomia Questionnaire (XQ)[89]
Symptom burden	MD Anderson Symptom Inventory Head and Neck Cancer Module (MDASI-HN)[90] Vanderbilt Head and Neck Symptom Survey (VHNSS)[91]

hydration, and medication, it does not eliminate the risk of aspiration and aspiration pneumonia.

Aspiration, a direct result of impaired airway safety, is a significant morbidity after treatment for HNC, which often places undue medical and nutritional burden on patients. Although the prevalence of aspiration is thought to be underreported owing to its silent nature (ie, silent aspiration, without cough or other symptoms), aspiration ranges from 7% to 31% among patients with primary oropharynx tumors.[17,22] Further, it is reported that 11% of these patients develop aspiration pneumonia[21] and 4% are chronically dependent on a feeding tube after CRT.[23] Surveillance, Epidemiology, and End Results-Medicare data suggest also that the lifetime risk of developing aspiration pneumonia after CRT for oral cavity or oropharyngeal cancer approximates 20% to 25%, and this represents a 3-fold greater risk over noncancer controls.[98]

SUMMARY

This article provides a framework for proactive speech–language pathology services in assessment and treatment of patients with HNC. It is posited that speech pathology services initiate at diagnosis and continue throughout the continuum of survivorship. HNC and its oncologic treatment frequently disrupt speech and/or swallowing mechanisms, thus, adversely impacting an individual's health, functional status, and quality of life. Assessments of speech and swallow function help to guide decision making and expected outcomes. This is beneficial before and after medical intervention in an effort to guide plan of care, as well as rehabilitation and dietary plans. As discussed, assessment can also aid the maxillofacial professional to optimize fit and functionality of prosthetics for speech and swallowing. Intervention, both proactive (preventative) and reactive (after cancer therapy), assists in maintaining and improving speech and swallow function in the pursuit of improved quality of life. As such, speech–language pathologists are critical members of the multidisciplinary team who are responsible for the evaluation, patient education, treatment planning, symptom management, and rehabilitation of speech and swallowing. This article offers a framework for accurate diagnosis and evidence-based principals of rehabilitation for best practice to optimize the functional outcome of patients with HNC.

REFERENCES

1. Marur S, D'Souza G, Westra WH, et al. HPV-associated head and neck cancer: a virus-related cancer epidemic. Lancet Oncol 2010;11(8):781–9.

2. Deschler DG, Richmon JD, Khariwala SS, et al. The "New" head and neck cancer patient–young, nonsmoker, nondrinker, and HPV positive: evaluation. Otolaryngol Head Neck Surg 2014;151(3):375–80.

3. Fakhry C, Westra WH, Li S, et al. Improved survival of patients with human papillomavirus-positive head and neck squamous cell carcinoma in a prospective clinical trial. J Natl Cancer Inst 2008; 100(4):261–9.

4. Chaturvedi AK, Engels EA, Anderson WF, et al. Incidence trends for human papillomavirus-related and -unrelated oral squamous cell carcinomas in the United States. J Clin Oncol 2008;26(4):612–9.

5. Stenson KM, MacCracken E, List M, et al. Swallowing function in patients with head and neck cancer prior to treatment. Arch Otolaryngol Head Neck Surg 2000;126(3):371–7.

6. Starmer H, Gourin C, Lua LL, et al. Pretreatment swallowing assessment in head and neck cancer patients. Laryngoscope 2011;121(6):1208–11.

7. Pauloski BR, Rademaker AW, Logemann JA, et al. Pretreatment swallowing function in patients with head and neck cancer. Head Neck 2000;22(5): 474–82.

8. van der Molen L, van Rossum MA, Ackerstaff AH, et al. Pretreatment organ function in patients with advanced head and neck cancer: clinical outcome measures and patients' views. BMC Ear Nose Throat Disord 2009;9:10.

9. Strojan P, Hutcheson KA, Eisbruch A, et al. Treatment of late sequelae after radiotherapy for head and neck cancer. Cancer Treat Rev 2017;59:79–92.

10. Borras JM, Barton M, Grau C, et al. The impact of cancer incidence and stage on optimal utilization of radiotherapy: methodology of a population based analysis by the ESTRO-HERO project. Radiother Oncol 2015;116(1):45–50.

11. Kumar R, Starmer H, Alcorn E, et al. Radiation dose to the floor of mouth muscles predicts swallowing complications after chemoradiation in oropharyngeal squamous cell carcinoma. Int J Radiat Oncol Biol Phys 2013;84(3):S206–7.

12. M. D. Anderson Head Neck Cancer Symptom Working Group. Beyond mean pharyngeal constrictor dose for beam path toxicity in non-target swallowing muscles: dose-volume correlates of chronic radiation-associated dysphagia (RAD) after oropharyngeal intensity modulated radiotherapy. Radiother Oncol 2016;118(2):304–14.

13. Brennan PA, Bradley KL, Brands M. Intensity-modulated radiotherapy in head and neck cancer - an update for oral and maxillofacial surgeons. Br J Oral Maxillofac Surg 2017;55(8):770–4.

14. Petkar I, Rooney K, Roe JW, et al. DARS: a phase III randomised multicentre study of dysphagia- optimised intensity- modulated radiotherapy (Do-IMRT) versus standard intensity- modulated radiotherapy

(S-IMRT) in head and neck cancer. BMC Cancer 2016;16(1):770.

15. Hunter KU, Schipper M, Feng FY, et al. Toxicities affecting quality of life after chemo-IMRT of oropharyngeal cancer: prospective study of patient-reported, observer-rated, and objective outcomes. Int J Radiat Oncol Biol Phys 2013;85(4):935–40.

16. Goepfert RP, Fuller CD, Gunn GB, et al. Symptom burden as a driver of decisional regret in long-term oropharyngeal carcinoma survivors. Head Neck 2017;39(11):2151–8.

17. Hutcheson KA, Lewin JS, Holsinger FC, et al. Long-term functional and survival outcomes after induction chemotherapy and risk-based definitive therapy for locally advanced squamous cell carcinoma of the head and neck. Head Neck 2014;36(4):474–80.

18. Caudell JJ, Schaner PE, Meredith RF, et al. Factors associated with long-term dysphagia after definitive radiotherapy for locally advanced head-and-neck cancer. Int J Radiat Oncol Biol Phys 2009;73(2):410–5.

19. Francis DO, Weymuller EA, Parvathaneni U, et al. Dysphagia, stricture, and pneumonia in head and neck cancer patients: does treatment modality matter? Ann Otol Rhinol Laryngol 2010;119(6):391–7.

20. Wilson JA, Carding PN, Patterson JM. Dysphagia after nonsurgical head and neck cancer treatment: patients' perspectives. Otolaryngol Head Neck Surg 2011;145(5):767–71.

21. Hunter KU, Lee OE, Lyden TH, et al. Aspiration pneumonia after chemo-intensity-modulated radiation therapy of oropharyngeal carcinoma and its clinical and dysphagia-related predictors. Head Neck 2014;36(1):120–5.

22. Eisbruch A, Kim HM, Feng FY, et al. Chemo-IMRT of oropharyngeal cancer aiming to reduce dysphagia: swallowing organs late complication probabilities and dosimetric correlates. Int J Radiat Oncol Biol Phys 2011;81(3):e93–9.

23. Setton J, Lee NY, Riaz N, et al. A multi-institution pooled analysis of gastrostomy tube dependence in patients with oropharyngeal cancer treated with definitive intensity-modulated radiotherapy. Cancer 2015;121(2):294–301.

24. Colangelo LA, Logemann JA, Pauloski BR, et al. T stage and functional outcome in oral and oropharyngeal cancer patients. Head Neck 1996;18(3):259–68.

25. Borggreven PA, Verdonck-de Leeuw I, Rinkel RN, et al. Swallowing after major surgery of the oral cavity or oropharynx: a prospective and longitudinal assessment of patients treated by microvascular soft tissue reconstruction. Head Neck 2007;29(7):638–47.

26. Kreeft AM, van der Molen L, Hilgers FJ, et al. Speech and swallowing after surgical treatment of advanced oral and oropharyngeal carcinoma: a systematic review of the literature. Eur Arch Otorhinolaryngol 2009;266(11):1687–98.

27. Borggreven PA, Verdonck-de Leeuw I, Langendijk JA, et al. Speech outcome after surgical treatment for oral and oropharyngeal cancer: a longitudinal assessment of patients reconstructed by a microvascular flap. Head Neck 2005;27(9):785–93.

28. Lazarus CL, Husaini H, Anand SM, et al. Tongue strength as a predictor of functional outcomes and quality of life after tongue cancer surgery. Ann Otol Rhinol Laryngol 2013;122(6):386–97.

29. Kimata Y, Sakuraba M, Hishinuma S, et al. Analysis of the relations between the shape of the reconstructed tongue and postoperative functions after subtotal or total glossectomy. Laryngoscope 2003;113(5):905–9.

30. Seikaly H, Rieger J, Wolfaardt J, et al. Functional outcomes after primary oropharyngeal cancer resection and reconstruction with the radial forearm free flap. Laryngoscope 2003;113(5):897–904.

31. Futran ND, Wadsworth JT, Villaret D, et al. Midface reconstruction with the fibula free flap. Arch Otolaryngol Head Neck Surg 2002;128(2):161–6.

32. Hertrampf K, Wenz HJ, Lehmann KM, et al. Quality of life of patients with maxillofacial defects after treatment for malignancy. Int J Prosthodont 2004;17(6):657–65.

33. Schuster M, Stelzle F. Outcome measurements after oral cancer treatment: speech and speech-related aspects–an overview. Oral Maxillofac Surg 2012;16(3):291–8.

34. Kraaijenga SA, Oskam IM, van Son RJ, et al. Assessment of voice, speech, and related quality of life in advanced head and neck cancer patients 10-years+ after chemoradiotherapy. Oral Oncol 2016;55:24–30.

35. Lazarus CL. Effects of chemoradiotherapy on voice and swallowing. Curr Opin Otolaryngol Head Neck Surg 2009;17(3):172–8.

36. Starmer HM, Gourin CG. Is speech language pathologist evaluation necessary in the nonoperative treatment of head and neck cancer? Laryngoscope 2013;123(7):1571–2.

37. Pauloski BR, Logemann JA, Rademaker AW, et al. Speech and swallowing function after anterior tongue and floor of mouth resection with distal flap reconstruction. J Speech Hear Res 1993;36(2):267–76.

38. Furia CL, Kowalski LP, Latorre MR, et al. Speech intelligibility after glossectomy and speech rehabilitation. Arch Otolaryngol Head Neck Surg 2001;127(7):877–83.

39. Biazevic MGH, Antunes JLF, Togni J, et al. Survival and quality of life of patients with oral and oropharyngeal cancer at 1-year follow-up of tumor resection. J Appl Oral Sci 2010;18(3):279–84.

40. Dwivedi RC, Chisholm EJ, Khan AS, et al. An exploratory study of the influence of clinico-demographic variables on swallowing and swallowing-related quality of life in a cohort of oral and oropharyngeal cancer patients treated with primary surgery. Eur Arch Otorhinolaryngol 2012;269(4):1233–9.

41. Yang Z-H, Chen W-L, Huang H-Z, et al. Quality of life of patients with tongue cancer 1 year after surgery. J Oral Maxillofac Surg 2010;68(9):2164–8.

42. Smith BG, Hutcheson KA, Little LG, et al. Lymphedema outcomes in patients with head and neck cancer. Otolaryngol Head Neck Surg 2015;152(2):284–91.

43. Deng J, Murphy BA, Dietrich MS, et al. Impact of secondary lymphedema after head and neck cancer treatment on symptoms, functional status, and quality of life. Head Neck 2013;35(7):1026–35.

44. Skelly M, Spector DJ, Donaldson RC, et al. Compensatory physiologic phonetics for the glossectomy. J Speech Hear Disord 1971;36(1):101–14.

45. Skelly M, Donaldson RC, Fust RS, et al. Changes in phonatory aspects of glossectomy intelligibility through vocal parameter manipulation. J Speech Hear Disord 1972;37(3):379–89.

46. Hutcheson KA, Lewin JS. Functional assessment and rehabilitation: how to maximize outcomes. Otolaryngol Clin North Am 2013;46(4):657–70.

47. Knipfer C, Riemann M, Bocklet T, et al. Speech intelligibility enhancement after maxillary denture treatment and its impact on quality of life. Int J Prosthodont 2014;27(1):61–9.

48. Marunick M, Tselios N. The efficacy of palatal augmentation prostheses for speech and swallowing in patients undergoing glossectomy: a review of the literature. J Prosthet Dent 2004;91(1):67–74.

49. Irish J, Sandhu N, Simpson C, et al. Quality of life in patients with maxillectomy prostheses. Head Neck 2009;31(6):813–21.

50. Sullivan M, Gaebler C, Beukelman D, et al. Impact of palatal prosthodontic intervention on communication performance of patients' maxillectomy defects: a multilevel outcome study. Head Neck 2002;24(6):530–8.

51. Balasubramaniam MK, Chidambaranathan AS, Shanmugam G, et al. Rehabilitation of glossectomy cases with tongue prosthesis: a literature review. J Clin Diagn Res 2016;10(2):ZE01–4.

52. de Carvalho V, Sennes LU. Speech and swallowing data in individual patients who underwent glossectomy after prosthetic rehabilitation. Int J Dent 2016;2016:6548014.

53. Leonard R, Gillis R. Effects of a prosthetic tongue on vowel intelligibility and food management in a patient with total glossectomy. J Speech Hear Disord 1982;47(1):25–30.

54. Lee N, Puri DR, Blanco AI, et al. Intensity-modulated radiation therapy in head and neck cancers: an update. Head Neck 2007;29(4):387–400.

55. Nutting CM. Parotid-sparing intensity modulated versus conventional radiotherapy in head and neck cancer (PARSPORT): a phase 3 multicentre randomised controlled trial. Lancet Oncol 2011;12:127–36.

56. Murphy BA, Gilbert J. Dysphagia in head and neck cancer patients treated with radiation: assessment, sequelae, and rehabilitation. Semin Radiat Oncol 2009;19(1):35–42.

57. Lazarus C, Logemann JA, Pauloski BR, et al. Effects of radiotherapy with or without chemotherapy on tongue strength and swallowing in patients with oral cancer. Head Neck 2007;29(7):632–7.

58. Stinson SF, DeLaney TF, Greenberg J, et al. Acute and long-term effects on limb function of combined modality limb sparing therapy for extremity soft tissue sarcoma. Int J Radiat Oncol Biol Phys 1991;21(6):1493–9.

59. Lazarus CL. Management of swallowing disorders in head and neck cancer patients: optimal patterns of care. Semin Speech Lang 2000;21(4):293–309.

60. Watkin KL, Diouf I, Gallagher TM, et al. Ultrasonic quantification of geniohyoid cross-sectional area and tissue composition: a preliminary study of age and radiation effects. Head Neck 2001;23(6):467–74.

61. Awan MJ, Mohamed AS, Lewin JS, et al. Late radiation-associated dysphagia (late-RAD) with lower cranial neuropathy after oropharyngeal radiotherapy: a preliminary dosimetric comparison. Oral Oncol 2014;50(8):746–52.

62. Hutcheson KA, Yuk M, Hubbard R, et al. Delayed lower cranial neuropathy after oropharyngeal intensity-modulated radiotherapy: a cohort analysis and literature review. Head Neck 2017;39(8):1516–23.

63. Kulbersh BD, Rosenthal EL, McGrew BM, et al. Pretreatment, preoperative swallowing exercises may improve dysphagia quality of life. Laryngoscope 2006;116(6):883–6.

64. Carroll WR, Locher JL, Canon CL, et al. Pretreatment swallowing exercises improve swallow function after chemoradiation. Laryngoscope 2008;118(1):39–43.

65. Kotz T, Federman AD, Kao J, et al. Prophylactic swallowing exercises in patients with head and neck cancer undergoing chemoradiation: a randomized trial. Arch Otolaryngol Head Neck Surg 2012;138(4):376–82.

66. van der Molen L, van Rossum MA, Burkhead LM, et al. A randomized preventive rehabilitation trial in advanced head and neck cancer patients treated with chemoradiotherapy: feasibility, compliance, and short-term effects. Dysphagia 2011;26(2):155–70.

67. Carnaby-Mann G, Crary MA, Schmalfuss I, et al. "Pharyngocise": randomized controlled trial of

preventative exercises to maintain muscle structure and swallowing function during head-and-neck chemoradiotherapy. Int J Radiat Oncol Biol Phys 2012; 83(1):210–9.

68. Duarte VM, Chhetri DK, Liu YF, et al. Swallow preservation exercises during chemoradiation therapy maintains swallow function. Otolaryngol Head Neck Surg 2013;149(6):878–84.

69. Hutcheson KA, Bhayani MK, Beadle BM, et al. Eat and exercise during radiotherapy or chemoradiotherapy for pharyngeal cancers: use it or lose it. JAMA Otolaryngol Head Neck Surg 2013;139(11): 1127–34.

70. Virani A, Kunduk M, Fink DS, et al. Effects of 2 different swallowing exercise regimens during organ-preservation therapies for head and neck cancers on swallowing function. Head Neck 2015; 37(2):162–70.

71. Perry A, Lee SH, Cotton S, et al. Therapeutic exercises for affecting post-treatment swallowing in people treated for advanced-stage head and neck cancers. Cochrane Database Syst Rev 2016;(8): CD011112.

72. Manas A, Palacios A, Contreras J, et al. Incidence of oral mucositis, its treatment and pain management in patients receiving cancer treatment at Radiation Oncology Departments in Spanish hospitals (MUCODOL Study). Clin Transl Oncol 2009;11(10): 669–76.

73. Elting LS, Keefe DM, Sonis ST, et al. Patient-reported measurements of oral mucositis in head and neck cancer patients treated with radiotherapy with or without chemotherapy: demonstration of increased frequency, severity, resistance to palliation, and impact on quality of life. Cancer 2008;113(10):2704–13.

74. Logemann JA, Pauloski BR, Rademaker AW, et al. Swallowing disorders in the first year after radiation and chemoradiation. Head Neck 2008;30(2): 148–58.

75. Caudell JJ. Dosimetric factors associated with long-term dysphagia after definitive radiotherapy for squamous cell carcinoma of the head and neck. Int J Radiat Oncol Biol Phys 2010;76: 403–9.

76. Crary MA, Carnaby Mann GD, Groher ME, et al. Functional benefits of dysphagia therapy using adjunctive sEMG biofeedback. Dysphagia 2004; 19(3):160–4.

77. Carnaby-Mann GD, Crary MA. McNeill dysphagia therapy program: a case-control study. Arch Phys Med Rehabil 2010;91(5):743–9.

78. Crary MA, Carnaby GD, LaGorio LA, et al. Functional and physiological outcomes from an exercise-based dysphagia therapy: a pilot investigation of the McNeill Dysphagia Therapy Program. Arch Phys Med Rehabil 2012;93(7):1173–8.

79. Hutcheson KA, Barrow MP, Plowman EK, et al. Expiratory muscle strength training for radiation-associated aspiration after head and neck cancer: a case series. Laryngoscope 2018;128(5): 1044–51.

80. Arrese LC, Carrau R, Plowman EK. Relationship between the eating assessment Tool-10 and objective clinical ratings of swallowing function in individuals with head and neck cancer. Dysphagia 2017;32(1): 83–9.

81. Rogus-Pulia NM, Pierce MC, Mittal BB, et al. Changes in swallowing physiology and patient perception of swallowing function following chemoradiation for head and neck cancer. Dysphagia 2014;29(2):223–33.

82. Hutcheson KA, Lewin JS, Barringer DA, et al. Late dysphagia after radiotherapy-based treatment of head and neck cancer. Cancer 2012; 118(23):5793–9.

83. Chen AY, Frankowski R, Bishop-Leone J, et al. The development and validation of a dysphagia-specific quality-of-life questionnaire for patients with head and neck cancer: the M. D. Anderson dysphagia inventory. Arch Otolaryngol Head Neck Surg 2001;127(7):870–6.

84. Belafsky PC, Mouadeb DA, Rees CJ, et al. Validity and reliability of the eating assessment tool (EAT-10). Ann Otol Rhinol Laryngol 2008;117(12):919–24.

85. List MADAL, Cella DF, Siston A, et al. The performance status scale for head and neck cancer patients and the functional assessment of cancer therapy-head and neck scale. a study of utility and validity. Cancer 1996;1(77):2294–301.

86. Crary MA, Mann GDC, Groher ME. Initial psychometric assessment of a functional oral intake scale for dysphagia in stroke patients. Arch Phys Med Rehabil 2005;86(8):1516–20.

87. Jacobson BH, Johnson A, Grywalski C, et al. The voice handicap index (VHI) development and validation. Am J Speech Lang Pathol 1997;6(3): 66–70.

88. Rinkel RN, Verdonck-de Leeuw IM, van Reij EJ, et al. Speech Handicap Index in patients with oral and pharyngeal cancer: better understanding of patients' complaints. Head Neck 2008;30(7):868–74.

89. Eisbruch A, Kim HM, Terrell JE, et al. Xerostomia and its predictors following parotid-sparing irradiation of head-and-neck cancer. Int J Radiat Oncol Biol Phys 2001;50(3):695–704.

90. Rosenthal DI, Mendoza TR, Chambers MS, et al. Measuring head and neck cancer symptom burden: the development and validation of the M. D. Anderson symptom inventory, head and neck module. Head Neck 2007;29(10):923–31.

91. Murphy BA, Dietrich MS, Wells N, et al. Reliability and validity of the Vanderbilt Head and Neck Symptom Survey: a tool to assess symptom burden in

patients treated with chemoradiation. Head Neck 2010;32(1):26–37.

92. Gorenc M, Kozjek NR, Strojan P. Malnutrition and cachexia in patients with head and neck cancer treated with (chemo)radiotherapy. Rep Pract Oncol Radiother 2015;20(4):249–58.

93. Gellrich NC, Handschel J, Holtmann H, et al. Oral cancer malnutrition impacts weight and quality of life. Nutrients 2015;7(4):2145–60.

94. Meyer F, Fortin A, Wang CS, et al. Predictors of severe acute and late toxicities in patients with localized head-and-neck cancer treated with radiation therapy. Int J Radiat Oncol Biol Phys 2012;82(4): 1454–62.

95. McRackan TR, Watkins JM, Herrin AE, et al. Effect of body mass index on chemoradiation outcomes in head and neck cancer. Laryngoscope 2008; 118(7):1180–5.

96. Bhayani MK, Hutcheson KA, Barringer DA, et al. Gastrostomy tube placement in patients with oropharyngeal carcinoma treated with radiotherapy or chemoradiotherapy: factors affecting placement and dependence. Head Neck 2013; 35(11):1634–40.

97. Callahan CM, Buchanan NN, Stump TE. Healthcare costs associated with percutaneous endoscopic gastrostomy among older adults in a defined community. J Am Geriatr Soc 2001;49(11):1525–9.

98. Xu B, Boero IJ, Hwang L, et al. Aspiration pneumonia after concurrent chemoradiotherapy for head and neck cancer. Cancer 2015;121(8): 1303–11.

Nutrition and Perioperative Care for the Patient with Head and Neck Cancer

Amarbir Gill, MD, Donald Gregory Farwell, MD, Michael G. Moore, MD*

KEYWORDS

- Head and neck cancer • Malnutrition • Supplementation • Perioperative recovery
- Antibiotic prophylaxis • Anticoagulation

KEY POINTS

- Optimal recovery after major head and neck cancer surgery requires contributions from members of a multidisciplinary team. Preoperative counseling can facilitate preparation for surgery and recovery.
- Head and neck surgical wounds are often contaminated with flora from the upper aerodigestive tract. Appropriate perioperative antibiotic administration is needed to decrease the rate of wound infections.
- Perioperative pain management after major head and neck surgery is best accomplished through a multimodal approach that combines narcotic and nonnarcotic agents.
- Patients undergoing major head and neck cancer surgery are at increased risk for developing postoperative VTE and may require the use of sequential compression devices and/or systemic anticoagulants.
- Preoperative conditioning, incentive spirometry, early mobilization, intermittent positive pressure breathing, and deep breathing exercises can reduce the risk of pneumonia.

INTRODUCTION

The recovery from major head and neck ablative and reconstructive surgery is one of the more complex and challenging journeys patients and their families have to endure. The treatment will often have a significant impact on their ability to speak, swallow, and breathe. Because of the nature of their underlying malignancy, as well as the surgery associated with its removal, many individuals are at particularly high risk for perioperative complications, such as malnutrition, wound infections, VTE, and pneumonia. In addition, patients often battle pain and anxiety that can further predispose them to adverse outcomes. Herein, we summarize the current evidence-based best practices for the perioperative care of patients undergoing major head and neck surgery with the hopes of providing guidance that will improve outcomes.

PREOPERATIVE EDUCATION

Recovery after major head and neck surgery can be overwhelming for patients and families. Adjuncts such as tracheostomy and gastrostomy

Disclosure: The authors have nothing to disclose.
Department of Otolaryngology–Head and Neck Surgery, UC Davis School of Medicine, Sacramento, CA, USA
* Corresponding author. 2521 Stockton Boulevard, Suite 7200, Sacramento, CA 95817.
E-mail address: mgemoore@ucdavis.edu

Oral Maxillofacial Surg Clin N Am 30 (2018) 411–420
https://doi.org/10.1016/j.coms.2018.06.003
1042-3699/18/© 2018 Elsevier Inc. All rights reserved.

tubes, as well as wound care and drain management, require significant patient education and effort to optimize outcomes and avoid complications. Patients can benefit from preoperative education as a means to ease concerns and provide a smooth transition into the recovery period. Such teaching sessions have been shown to benefit patients in understanding the risks of operations, such as parotidectomy and thyroidectomy,[1] with shorter intervals between the education and surgery providing the most benefit.[2] Effective approaches include:

1. Patient education brochures,[3]
2. Preoperative visits with a social worker,[4]
3. Counseling sessions with a speech language pathologist (for patients preparing for total laryngectomy),[5] and
4. The use of multimedia and/or computer-based educational modules.[6,7]

Preoperative education is beneficial to patients undergoing major head and neck cancer surgery, and should be offered, when possible.

NUTRITION

Head and neck cancer and its associated therapy can significantly predispose patients to the development of malnutrition. Etiologies of malnutrition can include difficulty or pain with swallowing, loss of appetite/poor dietary habits, alterations in taste and saliva production, depression, and poor social support. In fact, malnutrition has been shown to occur in up to 50% of this population[8] and can have a significant negative impact on patient quality of life[9] and survival.[10]

For patients undergoing therapy for head and neck cancer, the identification and treatment of significant malnutrition is critical to improving outcomes. The optimization of perioperative nutrition has been shown to reduce the risk of wound infection and refeeding syndrome, and decrease duration of stay in patients undergoing surgical management of head and neck cancer.[11] A recent publication examined the impact of the Enhanced Recovery After Surgery, emphasizing the importance of nutrition on perioperative outcomes.[10] As a part of this effort, it is important to have close communication between all members of the multidisciplinary team, including surgeons and dietary/nutritional experts.

Patient Assessment and Screening for Malnutrition

The evaluation of a patient's nutritional and functional status allows for identification of modifiable factors that can in turn reduce morbidity and avoid interruptions in treatment. Although there are numerous tools that have been proposed for screening patients for clinically significant malnutrition, percent body weight loss and the validated Patient-Generated Subjective Global Assessment (PG-SGA) survey have demonstrated the most relevance.[11–14]

The most straightforward and widely accepted criteria for identifying severe malnutrition is the loss of 10% of body weight over a 6-month period or 5% of body weight over the past month. This is also the method endorsed by the National Comprehensive Cancer Network.[15,16] As a screening tool, when compared with well-nourished patients, this degree of weight loss has been shown independently to predispose individuals to major surgical complications,[12–14] a lower quality of life,[9,17] and increased mortality.[18,19] Van Bokhorst-de van der Schueren and colleagues[13] demonstrated that, after taking into account weight loss greater than 10% as a prognosticator of malnutrition and surgical complications, additional measurements, including percent ideal body weight, nutritional index, and serum albumin were not predictive of major complications. Gianotti and colleagues[14] similarly demonstrated that unlike weight loss of greater than 10%, albumin, total lymphocyte count, total iron-binding capacity, and serum cholinesterase showed a nonsignificant improvement in predictive ability of postoperative infection. In addition to weight loss, the PG-SGA has also shown application as a validated tool for the assessment of malnutrition in the population of patients with cancer (Fig. 1).[11,12]

The PG-SGA survey categorizes the patient into 1 of 3 nutritional categories, with the most severely malnourished category being predictive of surgical complications. Indeed, Ravasco and colleagues[12] compared the PG-SGA with percent body weight loss and body mass index in an attempt to identify the best prognosticator of malnutrition. The authors demonstrated that weight loss was the best single prognosticator, but sensitivity and positive predictive value could be improved by combining weight loss with the PG-SGA.

Summary
Percent body weight loss greater than 5% over the last month or greater than 10% over the last 6 months can adequately identify patients at greatest risk of postoperative complications from severe malnourishment. The addition of the PG-SGA may be able to identify a larger number of such patients.

Patient–Generated SGA* of Nutritional Status

History

1. Weight

In summary of my current and recent weight:

I currently weigh about _____ pounds

I am about _____ feet _____ tall

A year ago I weighed about _____ pounds

Six months ago I weighed about _____ pounds

During the past two weeks my weight has:

☐ decreased   ☐ not changed   ☐ increased

3. Symptoms

I have had the following problems that kept me from eating enough (check all that apply):

☐ no problems eating

☐ no appetite, just did not feel like eating

☐ nausea   ☐ vomiting

☐ constipation   ☐ diarrhea

☐ mouth sores   ☐ dry mouth

☐ pain; where? _____

☐ things taste funny or have no taste

☐ smells bother me

☐ other_____

2. Food Intake

As compared to my normal, I would rate my food intake during the past month as either:

☐ unchanged

☐ more than usual

☐ less than usual

I am now taking: ☐ little solid food
                    ☐ only liquids
                    ☐ only nutritional supplements
                    ☐ very little of anything

4. Functional Capacity

Over the past month, I would rate my activity as generally:

☐ normal with no limitations

☐ not my normal self, but able to be up and about with fairly normal activities

☐ not feeling up to most things, but in bed less than half the day

☐ able to do little activity and spend most of the day in bed or chair

☐ pretty much bedridden, rarely out of bed

THE REMAINDER OF THIS FORM WILL BE COMPLETED BY YOUR DOCTOR, NURSE, OR THERAPIST. THANK YOU.

5. Disease and Its Relation to Nutritional Requirements

Primary diagnosis (specify) _____

Stage, if known_____

Metabolic demand (stress):   ☐ no stress   ☐ low stress   ☐ moderate stress   ☐ high stress

Physical

For each trait specify: 0 = normal   1 = mild   2 = moderate   3 = severe

_____ loss of subcutaneous fat (triceps, chest)   _____ muscle wasting (quadriceps, deltoids)   _____ ankle edema   _____ sacral edema   _____ ascites

SGA Rating

Select one

☐ A = well nourished   ☐ B = moderately (or suspected of being) malnourished   ☐ C = severely malnourished

*SGA = Subjective Global Assessment   © 1995

Fig. 1. Patient-Generated Subjective Global Assessment survey. This tool can be used in the pretreatment assessment of patients for clinically significant malnutrition. (*From* Ottery FD. Definition of standardized nutritional assessment and interventional pathways in oncology. Nutrition 1996;12:S17; with permission.)

Perioperative Nutrition and Hydration Management

Although prior dogma dictated the avoidance of oral intake of food and liquids starting at midnight the night before surgery, more aggressive preoperative hydration and carbohydrate loading has been shown to be safe with no increase in aspiration rates when compared with more prolonged fasting.[20–22] Indeed, several studies have demonstrated that preoperative carbohydrate loading can improve perioperative outcomes. Presumably, this strategy works by minimizing catabolism and insulin resistance, thus providing better glucose control and maintenance of lean body mass.[21] However, although the safety of this approach has been confirmed,[22] appropriately controlled high-quality studies are needed to evaluate the efficacy of carbohydrate loading on duration of stay and perioperative outcomes.

The following are the currently accepted guidelines for preoperative hydration and carbohydrate loading.[20–22]

- Intake of solids are recommended up until 6 hours before general anesthesia, except in high-risk patients.
- All except high-risk patients should continue to consume clear liquids up to 2 hours before surgery.
- Between 2 and 4 hours before surgery, patients should consume a carbohydrate-rich (>50 g) clear liquid beverage.

Early Resumption of Postoperative Nutrition

For patients undergoing major ablative and/or reconstructive surgery of the upper aerodigestive tract, special considerations must be made for the postoperative initiation of nutrition. Such individuals may be at increased risk for wound breakdown owing to intraoral or pharyngeal repairs. Moreover, they often are prone to aspiration owing to alterations in their anatomy, sensation, swallowing physiology, and/or mentation in the immediate postoperative period. However, it has been demonstrated that early reinitiation of nutrition (ie, within 24 hours) after major surgery for cancer improves patient outcomes.[10] This goal can be accomplished via the resumption of oral intake (when there is a safe swallow and minimal to no violation of the upper aerodigestive tract), enteral tube feeds (via nasogastric or gastrostomy tube in individuals who have had major surgery of the oral cavity and/or pharynx and/or who are deemed high risk for aspiration), or parenteral nutrition (only to be used in circumstances where enteral feeding is not possible or safe).

Perioperative Nutrition in Malnourished Patients

Nutritional supplementation is recommended for patients found to have severe malnutrition on their preoperative screening. In their 2016 guidelines, Talwar and colleagues[23] recommend perioperative nutritional support for patients with a body mass index of less than 18.5 kg/m^2, weight loss

of greater than 10% body weight over last 6 months, PG-SGA grade C, serum albumin of less than 30 g/L, and inadequate intake (ie, <60% of caloric needs). Indeed, data demonstrate that the strongest evidence for supplementation is for patients with a greater than 10% weight loss in the last 6 months.[13,14] These authors also recommend initiation of nutritional therapy if the patient is unable to eat for more than 7 days. In these high-risk patients, both Talwar and colleagues[23] and Weimann and colleagues[24] recommend 10 to 14 days of preoperative supplementation. Findlay and colleagues[25] advocate for energy intake goal of 125 kJ/kg/d with close monitoring of postoperative weight.

Immune-Enhancing Nutrition

Several prospective cohort studies have suggested the superiority of immunonutrition (enteral feeds supplemented by a combination of arginine, omega 3, and RNA) over standard enteral nutrition; however, the quality of data is not sufficient to make definitive conclusions.[26,27] Riso and colleagues[26] examined 44 patients with head and neck cancer and demonstrated a significant decrease in postoperative complications and duration of stay among the cohort placed on immunonutrition compared with the patients consuming standard enteral feeds. Several randomized clinical trials (RCTs) were also performed comparing immunonutrition to standard enteral feeds in patients undergoing surgery for gastrointestinal cancer. Braga and associates[27] and Daly and colleagues[28] demonstrated a significant decrease in duration of hospitalization and postoperative complications among the immunonutrition cohort when successfully fed patients were analyzed. Conversely, the RCT performed by Schilling and colleagues[29] included 41 patients and failed to identify any significant difference in postoperative infections between the cohort receiving immunonutrition versus standard enteral therapy versus total parenteral nutrition.

Additionally, a review of 10 RCTs by Stableforth and colleagues[30] compared immunonutrition with standard enteral therapy in patients undergoing surgery for head and neck cancer. Their analysis revealed no significant difference in complications between the 2 groups. Nevertheless, the authors did demonstrate a 3.5-day decrease in duration hospital stay among the patients who received immunonutrition. The authors were unable to demonstrate the etiology of this observation and recommended additional, better powered RCTs. Finally, when implemented, immune-enhancing feeds should be used for 5 to 7 days preoperatively and at least 7 to 10 days postoperatively.[24,25]

Summary

The identification and management of severe malnutrition can significantly improve both short- and long-term patient outcomes. Moreover, although immune-enhancing nutrition has shown some benefit after cancer surgery, further study is needed to compare it with standard enteral nutrition and define its use in malnourished patients.

Indications for Feeding Tube Placement in Patients with Head and Neck Cancer

As discussed, patients with advanced head and neck cancer frequently suffer from weight loss and malnutrition. It is well-recognized that continued oral intake is critical in these patients. Prophylactic feeding tube placement is not recommended in patients without dysphagia at the initial assessment, because continued swallowing deterioration may develop from nonuse. Patients with preexisting dysphagia and those likely to develop dysphagia during their cancer therapy should be assessed and longitudinally followed by a qualified speech language pathologist with a goal of continued oral intake. There are patients, however, who are particularly high risk for severe dysphagia and/or malnutrition, where feeding tube placement should be considered.[15]

The decision between prophylactic and reactive feeding tube placement is of considerable importance to practitioners and patients.[31] Prophylactic feeding tubes are placed in individuals before the development of severe dysphagia with the goal of avoiding any treatment interruption that may develop when a swallowing difficulty progresses during therapy. Reactive feeding tubes are placed when a patient develops progressive dysphagia/malnutrition during or after treatment.

Advantages of prophylactic feeding tube placement:

- Placement does not require extra hospitalization over reactive feeding tubes and patients may experience less weight loss.
- Potential to avoid treatment interruptions owing to progressive dysphagia, dehydration and/or malnutrition.

Disadvantages of prophylactic feeding tube placement:

- When placed, gastrostomy tubes typically remain on average for 4 to 9 months.[31,32]
- Patients with gastrostomy tubes have been shown to have higher rates of perioperative wound/surgical complications.[31]

- Compared with a nasogastric tube, gastrostomy tubes may lead to longer feeding tube dependence, greater dysphagia, and an increased need for pharyngoesophageal dilation.[31,33]
- Longer gastrostomy tube dependence may lead to weakening and atrophy of pharyngeal muscles and worse recovery of swallowing function.[31,33]

Unfortunately, there is sparse literature looking at the benefit of feeding tube placement in avoiding malnutrition in patients undergoing major head and neck surgery. Placement in patients before head and neck chemoradiation therapy yielded an improvement of quality of life over those who received a reactive gastrostomy tube.[31,34]

Summary

Although the routine placement of a prophylactic gastrostomy tube is not recommended in patients undergoing surgery for head and neck cancer, it should be considered in certain high-risk individuals.

VENOUS THROMBOEMBOLISM PREVENTION

Patients undergoing surgery for head and neck cancer are at significant risk for the development of VTE. Studies have estimated that the general surgery population not receiving anticoagulation have a rate of DVT formation of between 15% and 30%,[35] which increases to 40% to 80% in those over 40 years of age with active cancer.[36] Patients with head and neck cancer are at significant risk of VTE because they often are frequent smokers, advanced in age, undergo prolonged surgeries, and often have significant periods of relative immobility postoperatively. An appropriate strategy is to perform a preoperative VTE risk assessment using previously validated tools such as the Caprini Score. This system allows patients to ultimately be grouped into the following risk categories: very low, low, moderate, and high risk. Based on this classification, anticoagulation recommendations range from early mobilization to use of sequential compression devices to sequential compression devices and heparin or weight-based low-molecular-weight heparin given subcutaneously.

Complicating the decision for appropriate perioperative anticoagulation is the fact that such patients often have large wounds and other high-risk bleeding sites, such as pharyngeal incisions and/or tracheostomies. For each individual patient, it is necessary to weigh the risk of VTE and bleeding complications.

Summary

All patients undergoing major head and neck cancer surgery should have their risk for VTE assessed and consideration should be made for prophylaxis using sequential compression devices, with or without pharmacologic therapy.

EARLY POSTOPERATIVE MOBILIZATION AND PULMONARY PHYSICAL THERAPY

One of the most critical aspects of the perioperative recovery after major head and neck surgery is encouragement of early postoperative mobilization as well as the implementation of an aggressive regimen for pulmonary physical therapy. Without such care, patients are at significant risk for the development of VTE, pneumonia, and pressure ulcers, leading to significant morbidity and potential mortality.

With regard to postoperative physical activity, it has been shown that early mobilization decreases the risk of pneumonia in patients undergoing free flap reconstruction of the oral cavity.[37] In other fields of surgical oncology, early mobilization protocols have also been found to decrease medical complications and length of stay.[38,39] The recent Enhanced Recovery After Surgery protocol after head and neck free flap surgery review advocates mobilization within the first 24 hours postoperatively, when deemed safe by the surgical team.[10]

In addition to early mobilization, further measures should be taken to minimize the risk of perioperative pneumonia. Tools such as incentive spirometry, intermittent positive pressure breathing, and deep breathing exercises have shown usefulness in individuals after abdominal procedures.[40] Although there is a paucity of literature directly evaluating the head and neck surgical population, it is likely that such regimens would be applicable to this group.

Summary

Early mobilization within the first 24 hours, when safe, and aggressive pulmonary therapy are recommended after major head and neck surgery.

Perioperative Antibiotic Prophylaxis

The appropriate use of perioperative antibiotics involves an understanding of the risks of perioperative infection and the potential for development of resistant infections or antibiotic-related complications (ie, allergic reactions or antibiotic induced infections, such as colitis). The head and neck literature demonstrates no role for perioperative antibiotics in wounds classified as clean.[41] Clean contaminated procedures (ie, transmucosal procedures), however, benefit from perioperative antibiotics, which have been shown to decrease wound complications across multiple RCTs.[10,41] A perioperative regimen should consist of a single dose of antibiotics within an hour before the initiation of surgery and should be extended for an additional 24 hours postoperatively.[10,41–45] Studies have not shown a significant decrease in infection rates with a longer course of prophylactic antibiotics or with topical decontamination or topical antibiotics in patients with head and neck cancer.[10,41–47] Multiple studies have shown strong evidence that perioperative antibiotics should cover gram-positives and anaerobes in this patient population; however, data on gram-negative coverage is more controversial.[48,49] Nevertheless, the head and neck literature most often recommends prophylactic coverage of gram-positive, gram-negative, and anaerobic bacteria.[44] Importantly, several studies have demonstrated increased rate of surgical site infection with the use of clindamycin.[50,51]

The American Health System Pharmacist recommends use of cefazolin/cefuroxime plus flagyl, or ampicillin-sulbactam, in clean-contaminated oncologic surgery in patients without a beta-lactam allergy.[52] In those patients with a beta-lactam allergy, the American Health System Pharmacist states that clindamycin may be used; however, these data demonstrate concern that clindamycin use may actually increase the risk of surgical site infections. Moreover, prior chemoradiation, clean-contaminated surgeries, immunosuppression, intraoperative blood loss, tracheotomy, prolonged operative time, and oral cavity cancer resections have been established as risk factors for surgical site infections.[53–56] Although many such factors are not modifiable, this information may be useful in patient counseling and risk assessment.

Summary

For head and neck surgery procedures that are classified as clean, no perioperative antibiotics are recommended. For clean-contaminated surgeries, 24 hours of perioperative antibiotics with gram-positive, gram-negative, and anaerobe coverage should be used. These antibiotics should be initiated within 1 hour before surgical incision. Additional patient and disease factors may impact infection risk and should be considered when determining the antibiotic regimen for a particular patient.

PAIN MANAGEMENT

Patients undergoing major head and neck oncologic surgery suffer from significant pain related to their surgical wounds. Adequately addressing this discomfort is critical to allow for appropriate resumption of activity. Various combinations of acetaminophen, nonsteroidal antiinflammatory drugs, opioids, gabapentin, and local anesthesia have been discussed in the literature. Acetaminophen has been shown to be an effective nonopioid analgesic agent for control of postoperative pain.[57] Although the intravenous route may demonstrate more reliable plasma levels,[58] intravenous administration has shown no advantage in pain control over oral administration[59] and is considerably more expensive.

There are good data demonstrating advantages of cyclooxygenase-2 inhibitors, such as celecoxib, on postoperative pain control across various surgeries, most commonly orthopedic and plastic surgery.[10,60–63] However, data have shown that both nonsteroidal antiinflammatory drugs and cyclooxygenase-2 inhibitors can increase risk of myocardial infarction, heart failure, and hypertension, which may be more pronounced in patients with preoperative risk factors, female gender, longer use of medication, and advanced age.[60,61] Celecoxib is the preferred agent in these situations, because it is the least likely to cause these adverse effects compared with other nonsteroidal antiinflammatory drugs and cyclooxygenase-2 inhibitors.[60,61] Wax and colleagues[64] demonstrated a lack of adverse effects of celecoxib on wound healing and free flap survival in a rat model. An additional advantage of celecoxib is that the mechanism of action does not inhibit platelet function and thus theoretically does not increase postoperative bleeding complications.[65] However, case reports have documented an association between use of celecoxib and bleeding after surgery.[66]

Gabapentin is a nonnarcotic medication that aims at addressing neuropathic pain. A single dose of the drug before tongue carcinoma resection and free flap reconstruction, when compared with controls, has been shown to significantly reduce postoperative pain scores, morphine requirement, or analgesia-related nausea and vomiting.[67] Moreover, Doleman and colleagues[68] performed a large metaanalysis of 133 RCTs comparing perioperative gabapentin (doses ranging from 200 to 1200 mg) with controls and demonstrated a significant decrease in postoperative pain scores and opioid requirements in the first 24 hours. Their metaanalysis also demonstrated that nausea, vomiting, and itching were decreased in this patient population and sedation was increased.[68] Most trials did not examine the long-term use of gabapentin on pain scores, but 8 trials did show improvement in chronic pain scores at 3 months postoperatively.[68] Patient satisfaction scores and preoperative anxiety were also significantly improved with the use of gabapentin compared with controls.[68] More research, including RCTs, is needed to validate the therapeutic effects of gabapentin in patients with head and neck cancer.

Data on the efficacy of local neuromuscular blockades in head and neck patients are very limited. A single study examining the effect of mandibular nerve block in patients undergoing oropharyngeal surgeries demonstrated improved analgesia.[69] A few studies have shown a significant effect on postoperative analgesia when bilateral superior cervical plexus anesthetic nerve blocks are performed for patients undergoing thyroidectomy with or without parathyroidectomy,[70] with a decrease in the duration of stay.[71] However, a large metaanalysis of RCTs analyzing these same blocks in patients undergoing thyroid surgery concluded that, although analgesia can be obtained, the results were not clinically significant.[72] Thus, additional research is necessary to further identify potential benefit of local neuromuscular blocks on postoperative analgesia in the patient population with head and neck cancer.

A multimodal approach to achieve postoperative pain control is recommended. The combination of opioid and nonopioid medications can optimize analgesia while minimizing sedation and allowing for early mobilization.

SUMMARY

Perioperative management of patients undergoing significant ablative and/or reconstructive surgery of the head and neck is complex. Successful care requires an organized and multidisciplinary approach to optimize the patient's recovery. Preoperatively, patients should be assessed for their surgical candidacy and educated on the risks and benefits and the functional and physiologic changes that may result from the procedure. Those patients who elect to pursue treatment should be screened for clinically significant malnutrition and managed appropriately. Around the time of surgery, adequate antibiotic and VTE prophylaxis should be provided based on the nature of the surgery and patient-specific risks. In the perioperative period, a multimodal approach to analgesia should be implemented, with aggressive resumption of postoperative activity and nutrition to minimize the potential for complications. Although the treatment for each patient should be individualized, these evidence-based principles can serve as a guide to help both clinicians and caregivers support those under their care.

REFERENCES

1. Chan Y, Irish JC, Wood SJ, et al. Patient education and informed consent in head and neck surgery. Arch Otolaryngol Head Neck Surg 2002;128:1269–74.
2. Adams MT, Chen B, Makowski R, et al. Multimedia approach to preoperative adenotonsillectomy counseling. Otolaryngol Head Neck Surg 2012;146:461–6.
3. Clarke LK. Pathways for head and neck surgery: a patient-education tool. Clin J Oncol Nurs 2002;6:78–82.
4. Yarlagadda BB, Hatton E, Huettig J, et al. Patient and staff perceptions of social worker counseling before surgical therapy for head and neck cancer. Health Soc Work 2015;40:120–4.
5. Shenson JA, Craig JN, Rohde SL. Effect of preoperative counseling on hospital length of stay and readmissions after total laryngectomy. Otolaryngol Head Neck Surg 2017;156:289–98.
6. Bollschweiler E, Apitzsch J, Apitsch J, et al. Improving informed consent of surgical patients using a multimedia-based program? Results of a prospective randomized multicenter study of patients before cholecystectomy. Ann Surg 2008;248:205–11.
7. Siu JM, Rotenberg BW, Franklin JH, et al. Multimedia in the informed consent process for endoscopic sinus surgery: a randomized control trial. Laryngoscope 2016;126:1273–8.
8. Bertrand PC, Piquet MA, Bordier I, et al. Preoperative nutritional support at home in head and neck cancer patients: from nutritional benefits to the prevention of the alcohol withdrawal syndrome. Curr Opin Clin Nutr Metab Care 2002;5:435–40.
9. Langius JA, van Dijk AM, Doornaert P, et al. More than 10% weight loss in head and neck cancer patients during radiotherapy is independently associated with deterioration in quality of life. Nutr Cancer 2013;65:76–83.
10. Dort JC, Farwell DG, Findlay M, et al. Optimal perioperative care in major head and neck cancer surgery with free flap reconstruction: a consensus review and recommendations from the enhanced recovery after surgery society. JAMA Otolaryngol Head Neck Surg 2017;143:292–303.
11. Ottery FD. Definition of standardized nutritional assessment and interventional pathways in oncology. Nutrition 1996;12:S15–9.
12. Ravasco P, Monteiro-Grillo I, Vidal PM, et al. Nutritional deterioration in cancer: the role of disease and diet. Clin Oncol (R Coll Radiol) 2003;15:443–50.
13. van Bokhorst-de van der Schueren MA, van Leeuwen PA, Sauerwein HP, et al. Assessment of malnutrition parameters in head and neck cancer and their relation to postoperative complications. Head Neck 1997;19:419–25.
14. Gianotti L, Braga M, Radaelli G, et al. Lack of improvement of prognostic performance of weight loss when combined with other parameters. Nutrition 1995;11:12–6.
15. Pfister DG, Spencer S, Adelstein D. Head and neck cancers, version 2 2018. Available at: https://www.nccn.org/professionals/physician_gls/pdf/head-and-neck.pdf. Accessed August 24, 2018.
16. Satyanarayana R, Klein S. Clinical efficacy of perioperative nutrition support. Curr Opin Clin Nutr Metab Care 1998;1:51–8.
17. Van Bokhorst-de Van der Schuer MA, Langendoen SI, Vondeling H, et al. Perioperative enteral nutrition and quality of life of severely malnourished head and neck cancer patients: a randomized clinical trial. Clin Nutr 2000;19:437–44.
18. Datema FR, Ferrier MB, Baatenburg de Jong RJ. Impact of severe malnutrition on short-term mortality and overall survival in head and neck cancer. Oral Oncol 2011;47:910–4.
19. Lim SL, Ong KC, Chan YH, et al. Malnutrition and its impact on cost of hospitalization, length of stay, readmission and 3-year mortality. Clin Nutr 2012;31:345–50.
20. Brady M, Kinn S, Stuart P. Preoperative fasting for adults to prevent perioperative complications. Cochrane Database Syst Rev 2003;(4):CD004423.
21. Pogatschnik C, Steiger E. Review of preoperative carbohydrate loading. Nutr Clin Pract 2015;30:660–4.
22. Bilku DK, Dennison AR, Hall TC, et al. Role of preoperative carbohydrate loading: a systematic review. Ann R Coll Surg Engl 2014;96:15.
23. Talwar B, Donnelly R, Skelly R, et al. Nutritional management in head and neck cancer: United Kingdom national multidisciplinary guidelines. J Laryngol Otol 2016;130:S32–40.
24. Weimann A, Braga M, Harsanyi L, et al. ESPEN guidelines on enteral nutrition: surgery including organ transplantation. Clin Nutr 2006;25:224–44.
25. Findlay M, Bauer J, Brown T, et al. Evidence-based practice guidelines for the nutritional management of adult patients with head and neck cancer. Sydney (Australia): Cancer Council Australia; 2015. Available at: http://wiki.cancer.org.au/australia/COSA:Head_and_neck_cancer_nutrition_guidelines.
26. Riso S, Aluffi P, Brugnani M, et al. Postoperative enteral immunonutrition in head and neck cancer patients. Clin Nutr 2000;19:407–12.
27. Braga M, Wischmeyer PE, Drover J, et al. Clinical evidence for pharmaconutrition in major elective surgery. JPEN J Parenter Enteral Nutr 2013;37:66S–72S.
28. Daly JM, Lieberman MD, Goldfine J, et al. Enteral nutrition with supplemental arginine, RNA, and

omega-3 fatty acids in patients after operation: immunologic, metabolic, and clinical outcome. Surgery 1992;112:56–67.

29. Schilling J, Vranjes N, Fierz W, et al. Clinical outcome and immunology of postoperative arginine, omega-3 fatty acids, and nucleotide-enriched enteral feeding: a randomized prospective comparison with standard enteral and low calorie/low fat i.v. solutions. Nutrition 1996;12:423–9.

30. Stableforth WD, Thomas S, Lewis SJ. A systematic review of the role of immunonutrition in patients undergoing surgery for head and neck cancer. Int J Oral Maxillofac Surg 2009;38:103–10.

31. Locher JL, Bonner JA, Carroll WR, et al. Prophylactic percutaneous endoscopic gastrostomy tube placement in treatment of head and neck cancer: a comprehensive review and call for evidence-based medicine. JPEN J Parenter Enteral Nutr 2011;35:365–74.

32. Lawson JD, Gaultney J, Saba N, et al. Percutaneous feeding tubes in patients with head and neck cancer: rethinking prophylactic placement for patients undergoing chemoradiation. Am J Otolaryngol 2009;30:244–9.

33. Mekhail TM, Adelstein DJ, Rybicki LA, et al. Enteral nutrition during the treatment of head and neck carcinoma: is a percutaneous endoscopic gastrostomy tube preferable to a nasogastric tube? Cancer 2001;91:1785–90.

34. Salas S, Baumstarck-Barrau K, Alfonsi M, et al. Impact of the prophylactic gastrostomy for unresectable squamous cell head and neck carcinomas treated with radio-chemotherapy on quality of life: prospective randomized trial. Radiother Oncol 2009;93:503–9.

35. Khorana AA. Risk assessment and prophylaxis for VTE in cancer patients. J Natl Compr Canc Netw 2011;9:789–97.

36. Agnelli G. Prevention of venous thromboembolism in surgical patients. Circulation 2004;110:IV4–12.

37. Yeung JK, Harrop R, McCreary O, et al. Delayed mobilization after microsurgical reconstruction: an independent risk factor for pneumonia. Laryngoscope 2013;123:2996–3000.

38. Jones C, Kelliher L, Dickinson M, et al. Randomized clinical trial on enhanced recovery versus standard care following open liver resection. Br J Surg 2013;100:1015–24.

39. Vlug MS, Bartels SA, Wind J, et al. Which fast track elements predict early recovery after colon cancer surgery? Colorectal Dis 2012;14:1001–8.

40. Thomas JA, McIntosh JM. Are incentive spirometry, intermittent positive pressure breathing, and deep breathing exercises effective in the prevention of postoperative pulmonary complications after upper abdominal surgery? A systematic overview and meta-analysis. Phys Ther 1994;74:3–10 [discussion: 10–6].

41. Busch CJ, Knecht R, Münscher A, et al. Postoperative antibiotic prophylaxis in clean-contaminated head and neck oncologic surgery: a retrospective cohort study. Eur Arch Otorhinolaryngol 2016;273:2805–11.

42. Carroll WR, Rosenstiel D, Fix JR, et al. Three-dose vs extended-course clindamycin prophylaxis for free-flap reconstruction of the head and neck. Arch Otolaryngol Head Neck Surg 2003;129:771–4.

43. Rodrigo JP, Alvarez JC, Gómez JR, et al. Comparison of three prophylactic antibiotic regimens in clean-contaminated head and neck surgery. Head Neck 1997;19:188–93.

44. Simo R, French G. The use of prophylactic antibiotics in head and neck oncological surgery. Curr Opin Otolaryngol Head Neck Surg 2006;14:55–61.

45. Liu SA, Tung KC, Shiao JY, et al. Preliminary report of associated factors in wound infection after major head and neck neoplasm operations–does the duration of prophylactic antibiotic matter? J Laryngol Otol 2008;122:403–8.

46. Simons JP, Johnson JT, Yu VL, et al. The role of topical antibiotic prophylaxis in patients undergoing contaminated head and neck surgery with flap reconstruction. Laryngoscope 2001;111:329–35.

47. Shuman AG, Shuman EK, Hauff SJ, et al. Preoperative topical antimicrobial decolonization in head and neck surgery. Laryngoscope 2012;122:2454–60.

48. Weber RS, Raad I, Frankenthaler R, et al. Ampicillin-sulbactam vs clindamycin in head and neck oncologic surgery. The need for gram-negative coverage. Arch Otolaryngol Head Neck Surg 1992;118:1159–63.

49. Skitarelić N, Morović M, Manestar D. Antibiotic prophylaxis in clean-contaminated head and neck oncological surgery. J Craniomaxillofac Surg 2007;35:15–20.

50. Mitchell RM, Mendez E, Schmitt NC, et al. Antibiotic prophylaxis in patients undergoing head and neck free flap reconstruction. JAMA Otolaryngol Head Neck Surg 2015;141:1096–103.

51. Pool C, Kass J, Spivack J, et al. Increased surgical site infection rates following clindamycin use in head and neck free tissue transfer. Otolaryngol Head Neck Surg 2016;154:272–8.

52. Bratzler DW, Dellinger EP, Olsen KM, et al. Clinical practice guidelines for antimicrobial prophylaxis in surgery. Surg Infect (Larchmt) 2013;14:73–156.

53. Park SY, Kim MS, Eom JS, et al. Risk factors and etiology of surgical site infection after radical neck dissection in patients with head and neck cancer. Korean J Intern Med 2016;31:162–9.

54. Anaya DA, Cormier JN, Xing Y, et al. Development and validation of a novel stratification tool for

identifying cancer patients at increased risk of surgical site infection. Ann Surg 2012;255:134–9.

55. Hirakawa H, Hasegawa Y, Hanai N, et al. Surgical site infection in clean-contaminated head and neck cancer surgery: risk factors and prognosis. Eur Arch Otorhinolaryngol 2013;270:1115–23.

56. Ogihara H, Takeuchi K, Majima Y. Risk factors of postoperative infection in head and neck surgery. Auris Nasus Larynx 2009;36:457–60.

57. Barden J, Edwards J, Moore A, et al. Single dose oral paracetamol (acetaminophen) for postoperative pain. Cochrane Database Syst Rev 2004;1: CD004602.

58. Jarde OBE. Parenteral vs oral route increases paracetamol efficacy. Clin Drug Investig 2013;110(3): 432–7.

59. Jibril F, Sharaby S, Mohamed A, et al. Intravenous versus oral acetaminophen for pain: systematic review of current evidence to support clinical decision-making. Can J Hosp Pharm 2015;68:238–47.

60. Aynehchi BB, Cerrati EW, Rosenberg DB. The efficacy of oral celecoxib for acute postoperative pain in face-lift surgery. JAMA Facial Plast Surg 2014; 16:306–9.

61. Derry S, Moore RA. Single dose oral celecoxib for acute postoperative pain in adults. Cochrane Database Syst Rev 2012;(3):CD004233.

62. Moodley I. Review of the cardiovascular safety of COXIBs compared to NSAIDS. Cardiovasc J Afr 2008;19:102–7.

63. Turajane T, Wongbunnak R, Patcharatrakul T, et al. Gastrointestinal and cardiovascular risk of nonselective NSAIDs and COX-2 inhibitors in elderly patients with knee osteoarthritis. J Med Assoc Thai 2009;92(Suppl 6):S19–26.

64. Wax MK, Reh DD, Levack MM. Effect of celecoxib on fasciocutaneous flap survival and revascularization. Arch Facial Plast Surg 2007;9:120–4.

65. Scott WW, Levy M, Rickert KL, et al. Assessment of common nonsteroidal anti-inflammatory medications by whole blood aggregometry: a clinical evaluation for the perioperative setting. World Neurosurg 2014;82(5):e633–8.

66. Stammschulte T, Brune K, Brack A, et al. [Unexpected hemorrhage complications in association with celecoxib. Spontaneously reported case series after perioperative pain treatment in gynecological operations]. Anaesthesist 2014;63:958–60.

67. Chiu TW, Leung CC, Lau EY, et al. Analgesic effects of preoperative gabapentin after tongue reconstruction with the anterolateral thigh flap. Hong Kong Med J 2012;18:30–4.

68. Doleman B, Heinink TP, Read DJ, et al. A systematic review and meta-regression analysis of prophylactic gabapentin for postoperative pain. Anaesthesia 2015;70:1186–204.

69. Plantevin F, Pascal J, Morel J, et al. Effect of mandibular nerve block on postoperative analgesia in patients undergoing oropharyngeal carcinoma surgery under general anaesthesia. Br J Anaesth 2007;99:708–12.

70. Egan RJ, Hopkins JC, Beamish AJ, et al. Randomized clinical trial of intraoperative superficial cervical plexus block versus incisional local anaesthesia in thyroid and parathyroid surgery. Br J Surg 2013; 100:1732–8.

71. Shih ML, Duh QY, Hsieh CB, et al. Bilateral superficial cervical plexus block combined with general anesthesia administered in thyroid operations. World J Surg 2010;34:2338–43.

72. Warschkow R, Tarantino I, Jensen K, et al. Bilateral superficial cervical plexus block in combination with general anesthesia has a low efficacy in thyroid surgery: a meta-analysis of randomized controlled trials. Thyroid 2012;22:44–52.

Imaging of Patients with Head and Neck Cancer
From Staging to Surveillance

Daniel P. Seeburg, MD, PhD[a],*, Aaron H. Baer, MD[a],
Nafi Aygun, MD[b]

KEYWORDS

- Imaging • Head and neck cancer • Staging • Surveillance • Squamous cell carcinoma
- FDG-PET/CT • MRI • CT

KEY POINTS

- Imaging is an integral part of staging, treatment planning, and surveillance of patients with head and neck cancer.
- New and improving imaging technologies increase accuracy of imaging studies but leave ordering providers with increased complexity in choosing the best study for a given indication.
- This review hopes to provide a summary of the latest imaging methods and recommendations for each of the various steps in managing patients with head and neck cancer.

INTRODUCTION

Few patients with head and neck cancer go through diagnosis, staging, treatment, and surveillance without at least one imaging study to aid in each one of these steps. With the availability of new and improving imaging technologies, including dual-energy computed tomography (CT), diffusion-weighted MRI, CT/MRI perfusion, and PET/MRI, it is becoming increasingly complex for the head and neck surgeon, radiation oncologist, or medical oncologist to request the most appropriate study for the specific indication at hand. This review hopes to provide a summary of the latest imaging methods and imaging recommendations for each of the various steps along the clinical path of patients with head and neck cancer, from initial staging to posttreatment surveillance. Because staging of head and neck cancer is different for various subsites of the head and neck, imaging is also discussed separately for

each. A separate discussion of imaging of perineural spread, imaging in the setting of an occult primary tumor, and imaging of lymph nodes is followed by a discussion of paradigms for surveillance imaging in the posttreatment neck.

ORAL CAVITY

The oral cavity extends from the lips anteriorly to the anterior tonsillar pillars and circumvallate papillae posteriorly. Squamous cell carcinoma (SCC) is by far the most common cancer of the oral region and makes up greater than 90% of all cancers there.[1] Common subsites include the floor of the mouth, oral tongue, gingiva, and buccal mucosa. SCC in the oral cavity and elsewhere in the head and neck is staged based on the tumor, node, metastasis (TNM) system developed by the American Joint Committee on Cancer (AJCC).[2]

CT and MRI are both commonly used for assessing the primary tumor site.[3,4] CT should

---

Disclosure Statement: The authors have nothing to disclose.
[a] Section of Neuroradiology, Charlotte Radiology, 1705 East Boulevard, Charlotte, NC 28203, USA; [b] Division of Neuroradiology, Johns Hopkins University, School of Medicine, 600 North Wolfe Street Phipps B100, Baltimore, MD 21287, USA
* Corresponding author.
E-mail address: daniel.seeburg@charlotteradiology.com

Oral Maxillofacial Surg Clin N Am 30 (2018) 421–433
https://doi.org/10.1016/j.coms.2018.06.004

be performed with intravenous contrast material (contrast-enhanced CT [CECT]) to increase tumor conspicuity. MRI has superior soft tissue contrast compared with CT and may provide a better assessment of smaller tumors and adjacent soft tissue invasion.[5] A common limitation in the oral region is streak artifact from dental restoration amalgam and beam hardening from adjacent mandible and maxilla. In this setting, MRI shows increased sensitivity for primary tumor detection over conventional CT.[3] However, newer CT technologies have contributed to significant improvements in metal artifact reduction. Dual-energy CT allows reduction of metal artifacts with virtual mono-energetic reconstructions at high kilo-electron volt levels.[6,7] In addition, new iterative software algorithms including iterative metal artifact reduction (IMAR) have further contributed to improved metal artifact reduction on CT, with the combination of IMAR and dual energy appearing to provide the greatest metal artifact reduction (**Fig. 1**).[8]

The decision of which modality to use ultimately needs to be tailored to the individual patient, taking into account such factors as dental artifacts, availability of the newer CT technologies for metal artifact reduction, the patient's ability to hold still (degradation of magnetic resonance [MR] images with tongue and swallowing movements), and the size of the primary tumor. In general, given the common artifacts in this region, the opinion of these authors is that MRI is preferred over CECT. However, when the primary tumor is small and superficial, allowing a thorough clinical assessment of extent, CT may be a more cost-effective choice for the evaluation of nodal basins. Per the National Comprehensive Cancer Network's (NCCN) guidelines, ^{18}F-fluorodeoxyglucose (FDG)- PET/CT may be additionally considered for stage III to IV (eg, T3 or N1) disease, as it may result in upstaging of disease.[9]

The primary tumor should be assessed for tumor size, deep (submucosal) extension, bone invasion, and precise characterization of adjacent structures involved, with special attention to structures delineated in the AJCC's guidelines for TNM staging. Second primary cancers are also important to identify during initial staging and on follow up surveillance imaging.[10] These can be either synchronous (discovered within 6 months of the first lesion) or more commonly metachronous. Most common locations for second primary malignancies are in the upper aerodigestive tract and lung. Nodal spread occurs primarily in neck levels I, II, and III.

Oral cavity malignancies have a high incidence of bone invasion, ranging from 12% to 56%[11]; but there is continued controversy in the literature over which modality is best for its detection. CT is generally considered superior for detection of subtle cortical erosion (using thin-section bone kernel images), but MRI is more sensitive for the

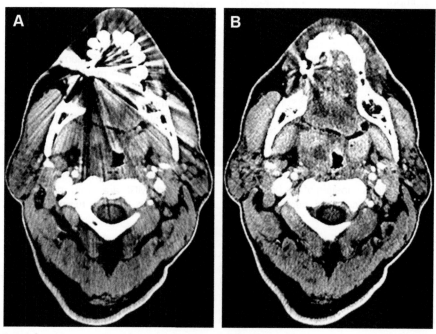

Fig. 1. IMAR. Axial noncontrast CT without (A) and with (B) IMAR in a patient with a necrotic right tonsillar mass.

identification of early marrow invasion. MRI may show marrow replacement without cortical disruption, so CT and MRI may be considered complementary for the assessment of bone involvement.[3] Reported sensitivity and specificity for detecting bone involvement by CT and MRI vary considerably[11–14] but are quite high (typically 80%–90%) and not statistically significantly different between these modalities. False-positive marrow signal changes on MRI can be seen with prior irradiation, osteoradionecrosis, and odontogenic infections (**Box 1**).

PHARYNX

The pharynx is located posterior to the nasal and oral cavities and extends from the skull base to the level of the cricoid cartilage. It is traditionally divided into the nasopharynx, extending from the skull base to the soft palate; the oropharynx, extending between the soft palate and hyoid bone; and the hypopharynx, below the hyoid bone to the caudal margin of the cricoid cartilage or top of the cricopharyngeus muscle. The mucosal surfaces of the pharynx are exposed to environmental risk factors for cancer development, especially alcohol and tobacco smoke, which has led to the concept of the condemned mucosa, consisting of widespread molecular and clinical changes. Clinically, this manifests as an increased risk for SCC of the head and neck, lungs, and esophagus. In addition, patients who develop SCC are at a lifelong increased risk of second primary malignancies of the aerodigestive tract.[16] Having a second primary malignancy confers decreased survival in those patients,[16] which argues for vigilant clinical and, potentially, imaging surveillance. Next, the authors discuss imaging considerations specific to the nasopharynx, oropharynx, and hypopharynx.

Nasopharynx

Nasopharyngeal carcinoma (NPC) is the most common type of malignancy in the nasopharynx, representing about 70% of neoplasms in this region. NPC comprises keratinizing carcinoma, nonkeratinizing carcinoma, and basaloid SCC. The nonkeratinizing type has a strong association with Epstein-Barr virus and is very sensitive to radiation therapy.[17] Lymphoma is the second most common malignancy in the nasopharynx, comprising about 20% of malignant tumors. Unlike NPC, lymphoma of the nasopharynx tends to arise in the midline and tends to expand the marrow of the clivus in the setting of skull base invasion.[18]

Cervical lymphadenopathy is the most common form of presentation, independent of tumor size, and is more pronounced than for other head and neck malignancies. This circumstance is reflected in the AJCC's staging of NPC, in which N1 disease is limited to lymph nodes measuring up to 6 cm in greatest dimension, compared with other cancers of the head and neck, in which the cutoff is 3 cm. Other presenting signs and symptoms include serous otitis media from eustachian tube dysfunction, trismus from masticator space invasion, headache from skull base invasion, and neuropathy from cavernous sinus invasion.[17]

The principal role of imaging is in mapping the extent of disease, particularly with regard to local extension and cervical metastases (**Box 2**). MRI is superior to CT for detecting early bone marrow infiltration, dural and intracranial involvement, and perineural spread. It is, therefore, considered the first choice for staging of NPC with or without additional CT.[9,19] Nodal spread is initially to retropharyngeal or level IIB nodes. NPC has a relatively high propensity for distant metastatic spread, including to bone, liver, and lung.[20] Per the NCCN's guidelines, assessment for distant

---

Box 1
Imaging of oral cavity tumors

- The best modality is CECT or MRI with and without contrast of the oral cavity and neck; CECT is preferred in the setting of motion artifact; MRI is overall preferred, especially in the setting of dental amalgam artifact.

- In the setting of dental amalgam artifact, use dual-energy CT with metal artifact reduction or MRI.

- For bone invasion, CT is superior for subtle cortical erosion; MRI is superior for early marrow invasion; CT and MRI may be considered complementary studies.

- Consider FDG-PET/CT for stage III to IV disease.

Box 2
Imaging of nasopharyngeal tumors

- The best modality is MRI with and without contrast of skull base to clavicle.

- For bone invasion, consider adding CT for equivocal cases of cortical erosion.

- Consider FDG-PET/CT for stage III to IV disease, N2-3 disease, and to assess for distant metastases, especially for nonkeratinizing histology, endemic phenotype.

metastases with FDG-PET/CT and/or chest CECT may be considered for any stage III or IV disease but especially for nonkeratinizing histology, endemic phenotype, or N2-3 disease.[9]

Because of its proximity to the skull base and pattern of spread, NPC is typically not treated with surgery but rather radiation therapy with or without chemotherapy.[9] After completion of definitive therapy, in the setting of clinical response to treatment, a posttreatment baseline MRI should be performed at 8 to 12 weeks (+/− PET) to serve as a comparison for any future studies. If there was involvement of the parapharyngeal space, pterygopalatine fossa, orbits, or skull base on the staging examination, it is not uncommon for some degree of abnormal MR signal to persist after treatment, sometimes indefinitely. The primary mass should, however, show significant decrease in size; there should be no residual enlarged lymph nodes (**Fig. 2**).[18]

Oropharynx

The oropharynx is located posterior to the oral cavity. Its anterior border is the circumvallate papillae of the tongue and the anterior tonsillar pillars. It includes the base of tongue, palatine tonsils, posterior oropharyngeal wall, and soft palate. SCC is the most common type of malignancy in the oropharynx, with lymphoma, minor salivary gland tumors, and mesenchymal tumors encountered less commonly.[21] The principal risk factors include alcohol, smoking, and human papilloma virus (HPV) infection.[22] Presentation is most commonly with regional nodal neck masses,

nonhealing mucosal ulcers, otalgia, and odynophagia. Nodal dissemination of disease is typically first to ipsilateral internal jugular chain nodes, principally levels II and III, and retropharyngeal nodes.[21]

The workup involves biopsy of the primary site or fine-needle aspiration of the neck node and HPV testing, followed by imaging to characterize the extent of disease and nodal involvement. Imaging is with CECT and/or MRI with contrast of the primary site and neck. Chest CT may be considered for advanced nodal disease to screen for distant metastases and for select patients who smoke to screen for lung cancer. FDG-PET/CT may be additionally considered for stage III to IV disease, as it may result in upstaging.[9]

Involvement of the mandible constitutes T4a disease, and is important to identify as it may affect clinical treatment decision making. As discussed in the section on oral cavity cancers earlier, CT and MRI may be complementary in equivocal cases of bone involvement. The base of the tongue can be a challenging subsite to assess on imaging, as it is made up of dense musculature and lacks the fat planes that provide greater contrast to tumors in other subsites. In addition, patients often have prominent lingual tonsils that can either mimic or mask small base-of-tongue tumors. Correlation with direct visual inspection is, therefore, essential. Extension of tumor across the base of the tongue increases the risk of contralateral nodal metastasis. For small exophytic tumors, transoral robotic surgery may be used, whereas tumors growing into the tongue base are more amenable to chemoradiation. Evaluation of the inferior and

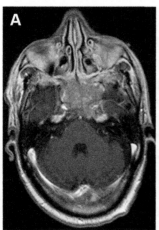 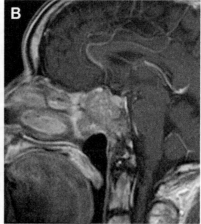 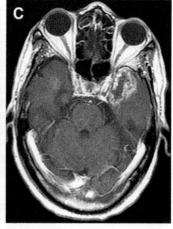

Fig. 2. Nasopharyngeal carcinoma. Axial (*A*) and sagittal (*B*) contrast-enhanced T1-weighted images demonstrate a solid enhancing nasopharyngeal mass invading the central skull base with obliteration of the sphenoid sinus. Axial contrast-enhanced T1-weighted image (*C*) approximately 18 months after completion of radiation therapy demonstrates resolution of the primary mass and interval development of an irregular rim enhancing mass in the left temporal lobe. This mass was radiation necrosis, a rare complication of radiation therapy.

posterior extent of base-of-tongue tumors is important because laryngeal involvement may impact clinical treatment between chemoradiation and surgery (pharyngolaryngectomy). The preepiglottic space of the upper larynx is located immediately beneath the vallecula and is bounded superiorly by the hyoepiglottic ligament. Invasion of this space by tumor can be assessed well with either CECT or MRI (**Box 3**).

Hypopharynx

As in the oropharynx and nasopharynx, most hypopharyngeal malignancy is SCC. Patients often present with advanced local disease, commonly with palpable cervical lymph node involvement. The subsites of the hypopharynx include the piriform sinus, postcricoid region, and the posterior hypopharyngeal wall. Most hypopharyngeal tumors are centered in the pyriform sinus. The apex of the pyriform sinus is typically at the level of the true vocal fold or cricoid cartilage, and its involvement with tumor portends a worse prognosis. These tumors can also rapidly spread into the larynx and can involve the cricoid or thyroid cartilage (T4a). Assessment of cartilage involvement can be challenging with imaging, and this is discussed at greater length later in the section on the larynx. Hypopharyngeal malignancies arising from the posterior hypopharyngeal wall are usually large and exophytic at presentation and may present with retropharyngeal nodes. An important imaging finding to make with these tumors is preservation of the prevertebral fat stripe between the tumor and prevertebral musculature, particularly well evaluated on MRI precontrast T1-weighted imaging. Although clinical evaluation during surgery remains the gold standard, this finding has a high negative predictive value in excluding invasion of the prevertebral fascia, which would increase the stage to T4b (**Box 4**).[23]

LARYNX

The larynx is made up of the supraglottic larynx, the glottis, and the subglottic larynx. The

---

Box 3
Imaging of oropharyngeal tumors

- The best modality is CECT or MRI with and without contrast of the oropharynx and neck.
- For bone invasion, CT and MRI may be considered complementary studies (see section on oral cavity).
- Consider FDG-PET/CT for stage III to IV disease.

Box 4
Imaging of hypopharyngeal tumors

- The best modality is CECT or MRI with and without contrast; MRI is especially useful in assessing for invasion of the prevertebral fascia; CECT is preferred in the setting of motion artifact—this area is prone to motion degradation.
- For cartilage invasion: consider dual energy CT (high sensitivity and specificity) or MRI with contrast (high sensitivity, modest specificity)
- Consider FDG-PET/CT for stage III to IV disease.

---

supraglottic larynx extends from the tip of the epiglottis to the level of the laryngeal ventricle. The glottis extends from the laryngeal ventricle 1 cm caudad and includes the anterior and posterior commissure at the level of the true vocal folds. The subglottic larynx extends below the glottis to the level of the lower margin of the cricoid cartilage. SCCs comprise most malignancies in this region.

Standard imaging of the larynx for both staging and surveillance is with CECT, which is faster and less prone to motion artifact than MRI. For the question of cartilage invasion, dual-energy CT and MRI may be of added benefit.[24] Cartilage invasion is critical to address during imaging evaluation of any laryngeal tumor, as this has important implications for staging and treatment.

On CT scans, the most reliable sign of cartilage invasion is through-and-through tumor spread with gross destruction of the cartilage and involvement of soft tissues beyond the outer cartilage margin. Lack of cartilage involvement can be suggested when the following 2 imaging findings are present: a continuous thin hypoattenuating line between cartilage and tumor and CT attenuation of nonossified cartilage that differs from that of tumor.[24] Unfortunately, nonossified cartilage frequently has CT attenuation very similar to that of tumors, making them almost indistinguishable. Sclerosis of the cartilage constitutes reactive change and does not necessarily mean that actual tumor invasion of cartilage has occurred. Overall, CT has a sensitivity of about 71% and specificity of 83% for detecting cartilage invasion.[25]

MRI has increased sensitivity of cartilage invasion of up to 96% with a corresponding high negative predictive value of up to 96%.[26] The shortcoming of MRI is its relative lack of specificity due to reactive inflammation, edema, and fibrosis in the vicinity of a tumor, which can lead to signal changes in the cartilage similar to those seen with tumor infiltration.[24] As a result, the specificity for thyroid cartilage invasion by MRI is only about 60%,[26] and the area of tumor extension into cartilage is more easily overestimated on MRI than CT.[24]

Dual-energy CT has the potential to increase the diagnostic performance and reproducibility for detection of thyroid cartilage invasion over conventional CT and MRI. Iodine from contrast material distributes into malignant tissue, but not into normal cartilage. By looking at iodine distribution images, a unique feature of dual energy CT, one can map the area of tumor taking up iodine. If this extends into cartilage contiguous with the tumor, cartilage invasion is likely. This approach increased the specificity over CECT from 70% to 96% in a recent retrospective study of 72 consecutive patients with laryngeal or hypopharyngeal cancer, without compromise in sensitivity (86% vs 86%).[27]

Extralaryngeal tumor spread constitutes T4 disease and, importantly, may occur without cartilage penetration.[28] Dual-energy CT images may facilitate the evaluation of extralaryngeal spread through the evaluation of iodine distribution maps alongside anatomic CT images (**Box 5**).[27]

NASAL CAVITY AND PARANASAL SINUSES

CT and especially MRI are the primary modalities used for imaging of the nasal cavity and paranasal sinuses. CT may be useful in the assessment of bony erosive change, including at the skull base. For staging of primary sino-nasal cavity malignancies, however, MRI with and without contrast is the best choice in assessing the extent of disease given its superior soft tissue contrast. Some of the malignancies encountered in this region include SCC, adenocarcinoma, minor salivary gland tumors, esthesioneuroblastoma, melanoma,

lymphoma, and undifferentiated carcinomas, including sino-nasal undifferentiated, small cell, and sino-nasal neuroendocrine carcinoma.[9,29] Nodal spread is typically to level I and II nodal stations as well as retropharyngeal nodes.

The principal role of the radiologist during staging is to assess the extent of tumor. Critical areas to evaluate for spread of tumor include the orbit, anterior cranial fossa, central skull base, and perineural spread (PNS). Important subsites of the naso-ethmoidal complex include left and right ethmoid complex, separated by the nasal septum, and 4 nasal cavity subsites (septum, floor, lateral wall, and vestibule). A major imaging challenge in staging these tumors is distinguishing tumor from adjacent inflammatory disease, especially with CT, given their similar attenuation levels. CECT can help, but MRI is superior given its better contrast resolution. Acute inflammatory secretions and mucosal thickening have high water content and are, thus, very bright on T2-weighted images. Tumors in this area, by contrast, are typically highly cellular, have relatively low intracellular and intercellular water content, and are, thus, intermediate in signal intensity on T2-weighted images.[30] Smaller field of view and thinner sections should be used for MRI of the face compared with MRI of the brain (**Box 6**).

Bony changes can help in characterizing tumors and in establishing a differential diagnosis. SCC typically causes aggressive bony erosion and destruction, often with only small bony fragments remaining. Metastatic carcinomas and some sarcomas and lymphomas can also cause aggressive bony destruction, although it is less common. In contrast, bony remodeling rather than destruction is more typical of schwannomas, inverted papillomas, most minor salivary gland tumors, lymphomas, esthesioneuroblastomas, some adenocarcinomas, and hemangiopericytomas (solitary fibrous tumors).[31]

SALIVARY GLAND TUMORS
Diagnosis

Ultrasound is a safe, cost-effective modality for identifying superficial submandibular and parotid

---

Box 5
Imaging of laryngeal tumors

- The best modality is CECT.
- For cartilage invasion, use dual-energy CT (high sensitivity and specificity) or MRI with contrast (high sensitivity, modest specificity).
- For extralaryngeal spread of tumor, use CECT or MRI; dual-energy CT may be of added benefit.
- Consider FDG-PET/CT for stage III to IV disease.

Box 6
Imaging of sino-nasal tumors

- The best modality is MRI with and without contrast of the face (including skull base) and neck.
- Consider FDG-PET/CT for stage III to IV disease.

space masses; but it is limited in visualization of the deep lobe of the parotid gland, and results are highly operator dependent. CECT is often the first-line imaging modality in adults with palpable salivary gland masses because it can usually distinguish between inflammatory/infectious and neoplastic causes. However, CECT may underestimate the lesion extent and is unreliable in distinguishing between benign and malignant tumors.[32,33]

MRI is currently the recommended modality for assessing tumor extent/infiltration, characterizing salivary gland tumors as benign or malignant, identifying perineural extension, staging, and assessing for postoperative recurrence. The MR features most specific for high-grade malignancy of the salivary gland include ill-defined tumor margins and signal hypointensity on T2-weighted imaging; together these two findings have a 70% sensitivity and 73% specificity for malignancy.[32,34] Benign salivary gland tumors are commonly well circumscribed, hyperintense on T2-weighted images, and are frequently in the superficial parotid lobe. Histopathologic analysis is often required for complete characterization, as there is substantial overlap between the MRI features of benign and low-grade malignant salivary gland tumors (eg, cystic changes and enhancement are common to both).[32] Advanced imaging techniques, such as diffusion-weighted MR, dynamic contrast-enhanced MR, and CT perfusion may improve diagnostic accuracy; but none currently obviate tissue sampling.[35–37]

FDG-PET/CT cannot reliably distinguish between benign and malignant salivary gland tumors, as benign salivary gland tumors (eg, most Warthin tumors) may be FDG avid.[37,38] Some tumors may be missed because of a relative high level of physiologic FDG concentration in normal salivary glands. There is probably a role for FDG-PET/CT in the detection of distant metastases, particularly with high-grade salivary gland tumors; but sensitivity for detection of metastases depends on FDG avidity of the primary tumor, and some malignancies (eg, adenoid cystic carcinoma) may be non–FDG avid.[38,39]

The value of fine-needle aspiration cytology in the preoperative diagnosis of parotid glad masses remains controversial with widely varying reports of sensitivity (between 41% and 100%) and specificity (between 86% and 100%).[40] A meta-analysis by Kim and Kim[41] reports that ultrasound-guided core needle biopsy of salivary gland masses yields a sensitivity of 94% and specificity of 98% with a low complication rate. Concern about tumor spread along the needle tract, although not substantiated by strong evidence, prevents widespread use of core biopsy.

Thus, preoperative fine-needle aspiration remains widely practiced, likely because of factors of convenience and perceived safety.

Staging and Prognostication

Staging of salivary gland malignancy is based on primary tumor size, local extent, invasion of adjacent organs, size and location of metastatic lymph nodes, and presence of distant metastases.[42] PNS is not included in staging criteria but is critical for prognostication and treatment selection, as it suggests aggressive tumor biology.[35] As in SCC of the head and neck, PNS is not uncommon in salivary gland malignancies and has been reported in 28% of cases of adenoid cystic carcinoma[43,44] (**Box 7**).

PERINEURAL SPREAD

PNS of tumor is a term that denotes macroscopic growth of tumor away from the primary site, along named nerves, and is detectable by imaging. In contrast, perineural invasion of tumor is a diagnosis made on histology, typically in a surgical specimen containing the primary tumor. All head and neck cancers can demonstrate PNS; but adenoid cystic carcinoma and, because of its high incidence, SCC are particularly commonly observed to show PNS. Basal cell carcinoma, melanoma, mucoepidermoid carcinoma, and lymphoma are also not infrequently found to have PNS.[45] PNS of head and neck cancers most commonly involves branches of the trigeminal and facial nerves and typically progresses from the primary tumor or surgical site afferently toward the central nervous system.

Imaging of PNS can be performed with CT or MRI, although MRI provides a better assessment of extent of disease due to its superior soft tissue contrast (**Box 8**). On CT, key imaging findings to

---

Box 7
Imaging of salivary gland tumors

- Best modality: MRI with and without contrast is ideal for assessing tumor extent, PNS, intracranial involvement, and locoregional recurrence.

- FDG-PET/CT has value in detecting FDG-avid distant metastases but is *not* superior to MRI for locoregional recurrence.

- MRI features most specific for parotid malignancy are as follows:

  ○ Ill-defined tumor margins

  ○ Low signal intensity on T2-weighted imaging

- Best modality: MRI with and without contrast of the skull base
- Most common head and neck malignancies with PNS
  - SCC of skin
  - SCC of mucosa
  - Salivary gland malignancy, particularly adenoid cystic carcinoma
  - Desmoplastic melanoma
  - Nasopharyngeal carcinoma
  - Basal cell carcinoma
  - Lymphoma and leukemia

look for are widening or erosion of skull base foramina or canals and obliteration of the normal fat density within the foramina or within the pterygopalatine fossa (PPF). On MRI, key imaging findings include nerve thickening and enhancement, loss of normal fat signal intensity within or around skull base foramina and the PPF, lateral bowing of the cavernous sinus, and replacement of the normal cerebrospinal fluid intensity within the Meckel cave (**Fig. 3**).

OCCULT PRIMARY CARCINOMA

Cervical lymph node metastases from an unknown primary tumor (CUP) constitute about 2% to 9% of all head and neck SCCs.[46] A meta-analysis of the diagnostic accuracy of FDG-PET/CT in the detection of primary tumors in patients with CUP found that the pooled detection rate, sensitivity, and

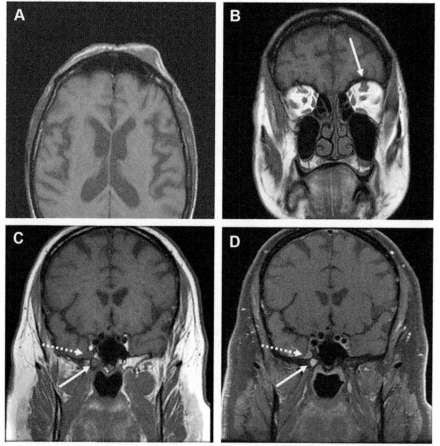

Fig. 3. Perineural spread. Axial noncontrast T1-weighted image (*A*) demonstrates a mass involving the left frontal scalp soft tissues. Coronal noncontrast T1-weighted image (*B*) demonstrates thickening along the expected course of the left frontal nerve (*white arrow*), a branch of V1 that supplies the forehead. Coronal T1 precontrast (*C*) and T1 postcontrast with fat saturation (*D*) images in another patient demonstrate thickening and enhancement of the right V2 segment within the foramen rotundum (*interrupted arrow*) and the right vidian nerve (*solid arrow*).

specificity were 37%, 84% (95% confidence interval [CI] 78%–88%), and 84% (95% CI 78%–89%), respectively.[47] In a prospective study comparing FDG PET/CT with CECT or combined CECT/MRI, Lee and colleagues[46] found that FDG-PET/CT was more sensitive (69%) in detecting primary tumors than either CECT alone (16%) or combined CECT/MRI (41%) in patients with CUP, whereas specificity was not statistically different between these modalities (**Box 9**). If nodal metastasis is shown to be HPV-positive SCC, then the occult primary is almost invariably in the oropharynx.

LYMPH NODES

The presence of regional nodal metastases is considered the single most important prognostic indicator in patients with head and neck SCC.[48] Imaging assessment of nodal metastases is unfortunately imperfect; only careful pathologic analysis of lymph nodes can be considered the gold standard of nodal involvement. The 2 major imaging criteria used for assessing nodal metastases are nodal size and the presence of central necrosis or nodal nonhomogeneity.

Using minimum axial diameter, jugulodigastric nodes (located in level IIA) are considered abnormal at greater than 11 mm and all other nodes at greater than 10 mm. A maximum longitudinal length to transaxial width ratio of less than 2 is suggestive of metastasis (indicating rounded configuration rather than the normal bean shape). For a group of 3 or more nodes in the drainage area of the primary tumor, one should suspect metastatic involvement if the minimum axial diameters are greater than 9 to 10 mm in level II or greater than 8 to 9 mm in the remaining neck.[21,49]

Irrespective of size, the most reliable imaging criterion for nodal metastasis is the presence of central necrosis. On CT, this manifests as a central area of low attenuation. On MRI, this manifests as a central area of T2 hyperintensity and central nonenhancement on T1-weighted postcontrast images.[21,49] Extracapsular spread (ECS) of nodal disease is associated with decreased survival. On CT, macroscopic ECS appears as an enhancing, often thickened nodal rim, typically with infiltration of the adjacent fat planes. The best radiologic predictors of pathologically proven ECS are central necrosis, irregular borders, and gross invasion of adjacent structures.[49,50] In a recent study of 111 consecutive patients with oral cavity SCC, central necrosis on preoperative imaging was found in 84% of patients with pathologically proven ECS but only in 7% of nodes without ECS.[50]

In patients with clinically and radiologically (CT/MRI) node negative (N0) necks, occult metastatic nodal spread is present in 20% to 40% of patients.[4] FDG-PET/CT improves the sensitivity and specificity of detecting metastatic lymph nodes over conventional CT and MRI, reducing the probability of occult neck metastases to 12% in one study.[51] However, the ability of FDG-PET/CT to detect small-sized metastatic lymph nodes remains limited, a limitation that is especially meaningful considering that more than 40% of metastatic cervical lymph nodes are less than 7 mm in diameter[52] and that most clinically N0 metastatic lymph nodes measure between 2 and 4 mm.[53,54] No imaging modality, including FDG-PET/CT, can replace the diagnostic capability of neck dissection for patients with N0 necks.[55] In the clinically and radiographically node negative neck, an elective neck dissection is typically performed based on the depth of invasion and location of the primary tumor.[9] Thus, FDG-PET/CT is not recommended for routine staging purposes of cancers of the head and neck that are stage 0, I, or even II.[9] FDG-PET/CT is, however, recommended in patients who appear to have stage III to IV disease, as it may alter management by upstaging (**Box 10**).[9,55]

SURVEILLANCE IMAGING IN THE POSTTREATMENT NECK
Imaging of Tumor Recurrence

Head and neck malignancies recur most commonly in the first 2 to 3 years after treatment. The most common sites of recurrence are in the operative bed and at the margins of the surgical site. Any new nodular or infiltrative soft tissue mass arising in or around the operative bed should raise suspicion for recurrent disease.[56,57] As the posttreatment neck can be difficult to evaluate

---

Box 9
Imaging for occult primary carcinoma

• Best modality: FDG-PET/CECT

Box 10
Lymph node evaluation

• The best modality is CECT or MRI with and without contrast.

• PET/CT is not routinely indicated in the clinically N0 neck.

• Consider FDG-PET/CT for stage III to IV disease.

on imaging because of the distortion of anatomy and postradiation changes,[56,57] it is critical to obtain high-quality baseline posttreatment imaging, especially for areas that are difficult to evaluate clinically, in order to have comparison images available for follow-up studies.[58]

MR perfusion and CT perfusion imaging are newer imaging techniques that show promise as tools to help differentiate recurrence from treatment change but are currently still being validated and not routinely used in many clinical centers. One possible use for MR perfusion imaging is in the context of equivocal FDG-PET/CT positive findings, to add specificity by further characterizing a lesion as recurrence or treatment effect. This technique may help obviate more invasive procedures, such as biopsy or surgery.[59]

Surveillance Imaging After Definitive Treatment

In general, after definitive treatment, patients enter a period of observation and surveillance. This period consists of regularly scheduled clinical examinations and typically involves repeating pretreatment imaging of the primary site (and neck, if treated) to establish a new baseline for comparison. CECT is a commonly used morphologic imaging modality for follow-up because it offers good assessment of pathologic cervical adenopathy and is rapidly acquired. MRI takes longer than CT to acquire and is more sensitive to artifacts from patient motion, repeated swallows, and rapid respirations, which are not uncommon in this patient population. However, as described earlier, for certain tumors that are close to the skull base, including nasopharyngeal carcinoma, as well as sino-nasal and salivary gland tumors, MRI is preferred because of its superior soft tissue contrast resolution and ability to detect perineural and dural invasion.[56]

Many studies point to the added benefit and value of adding FDG-PET to CECT for the initial baseline scan, which can impact decision-making, help predict prognosis, and serve as a cost-effective strategy to decrease the need for planned neck dissections.[60–62] For FDG-PET/CT, most studies suggest waiting at least 12 weeks after treatment, allowing enough time for immediate posttreatment change like inflammation and edema to abate but early enough to catch early recurrence or progression of disease.[61] There remains controversy over the routine use of FDG-PET/CT in surveillance of patients beyond the initial baseline scan at about 12 weeks.[60] Some particularly challenging posttreatment scenarios may, nevertheless, benefit from more long-term

surveillance with the addition of FDG-PET/CT, especially those with distorted anatomy and those that are difficult to evaluate clinically, for example, patients with oral cavity cancer requiring extensive resection and surgical reconstruction with tissue transfer. In this setting, FDG-PET/CT combined with CECT performed best in a retrospective study of detection of recurrent disease, compared with FDG-PET/CT without intravenous contrast or CECT alone.[63]

Interestingly, there is wide variation in self-reported routine surveillance FDG-PET/CT use among physicians who treat patients with head and neck SCC.[60] There has also been a general lack of accepted, data-driven consensus recommendations on the frequency and type of surveillance imaging, both in the surgical and imaging literature. As a response, the Head and Neck Imaging Reporting and Data System (NI-RADS) was recently developed for surveillance CECT with and without PET in patients with treated head and neck cancer.[64] This system was developed with multidisciplinary input from radiology; ear, nose, throat (ENT) surgery; and radiation and medical oncology. One possible surveillance imaging protocol is for the initial baseline scan to be performed at about 12 weeks after completion of definitive therapy with combined FDG-PET/CECT. If negative, a follow-up CECT of the neck and chest (without PET) is performed 6 months later. If that is also negative, a follow-up CECT of the neck (without PET) is performed 6 months after that, with continued spacing of surveillance CECT scans thereafter (**Box 11**). Thus, in this proposed protocol, only the initial baseline scan is a combined CECT and FDG-PET in the routine surveillance situation (**Fig. 4**).

Similar to primary tumors, it is assumed that detecting recurrent disease at a lower stage improves survival.[65] Greater frequency of imaging should, therefore, be performed early on, with gradual spacing over time. For low T-stage tumors without nodal disease that are easy to assess clinically, no routine surveillance imaging may be

---

Box 11
Surveillance imaging after definitive treatment

- Best modality: FDG-PET/CECT at 12 weeks; if negative, in 6 months CECT of the neck and chest; if negative, in 6 months CECT of the neck; if negative, continue to space further apart; MRI instead of CECT for sino-nasal cavity, nasopharynx, and SG tumors

- Use of NI-RADS for standardized reporting and management algorithms

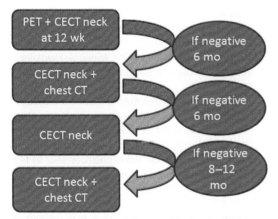

Fig. 4. NI-RADS. A possible surveillance imaging protocol after definitive treatment.

needed. Additional imaging outside of routine surveillance imaging should be performed as indicated based on worrisome or equivocal signs or symptoms.[9] Notably, most recurrences are reported by patients, so training patients to recognize suspicious signs and symptoms is also critical.[65]

There are several defined NI-RADS categories, each with linked recommendations, ranging from NI-RADS 1, no evidence of recurrence, to NI-RADS 4, known recurrent disease or definitive recurrence by imaging. A separate score is given to both the primary site and neck.[64,66] Initial performance of the NI-RADS system showed significant discrimination among categories 1 to 3 for predicting recurrent or persistent disease. The rates of positive disease were 3.8%, 17.2%, and 59.4%, for each of these NI-RADS categories, respectively, which included scans performed at the initial posttreatment time point of 12 weeks as well as later follow-up examinations during routine surveillance, with median imaging follow-up after the index scan of 51 weeks.[66] Overall, this is a promising new reporting template that has the potential to decrease variability in reporting within and across institutions, promote standardized management algorithms, correlate imaging with outcomes on a more granular level, facilitate data mining, and increase prognostic information of imaging at different time points after completion of therapy, which should be of value for patients and the entire clinical team involved in the care of patients.

REFERENCES

1. Palasz P, Adamski L, Goska-Chrzastek M, et al. Contemporary diagnostic imaging of oral squamous cell carcinoma – a review of literature. Pol J Radiol 2017;82:193–202.

2. Huang SH, O'Sullivan B. Overview of the 8th edition TNM classification for head and neck cancer. Curr Treat Options Oncol 2017;18(7):40.

3. Sarrion Perez MG, Bagan JV, Jiminez Y, et al. Utility of imaging techniques in the diagnosis of oral cancer. J Craniomaxillofac Surg 2015;43(9):1880–94.

4. Blatt S, Ziebart T, Krueger M, et al. Diagnosing oral squamous cell carcinoma: How much imaging do we really need? A review of the current literature. J Craniomaxillofac Surg 2016;44(5):538–49.

5. Kanda T, Kitajima K, Suenaga Y, et al. Value of retrospective image fusion of 18F-FDG PET and MRI for preoperative staging of head and neck cancer: comparison with PET/CT and contrast-enhanced neck MRI. Eur J Radiol 2013;82(11):2005–10.

6. Roele ED, Timmer VCML, Vaasen LAA, et al. Dual-energy CT in head and neck imaging. Curr Radiol Rep 2017;5(5):19.

7. Forghani R, Kelly HR, Curtin HD. Applications of dual-energy computed tomography for the evaluation of head and neck squamous cell carcinoma. Neuroimaging Clin N Am 2017;27(3):445–59.

8. Bongers MN, Schabel C, Thomas C, et al. Comparison and combination of dual-energy-and iterative-based metal artefact reduction on hip prosthesis and dental implants. PLoS One 2015;10(11): e0143584.

9. National Comprehensive Cancer Network. Head and neck cancers (Version 2.2017). Available at: https://www.nccn.org/professionals/physician_gls/pdf/head-and-neck.pdf. Accessed October 16, 2017.

10. Wong SJ, Heron DE, Stenson K, et al. Locoregional recurrent or second primary head and neck cancer: management strategies and challenges. Am Soc Clin Oncol Educ Book 2016;35:e284–92.

11. Handschel J, Naujoks C, Depprich RA, et al. CT-scan is a valuable tool to detect mandibular involvement in oral cancer patients. Oral Oncol 2012;48(4):361–6.

12. Vidiri A, Guerrisi A, Pellini R, et al. Multi-detector row computed tomography (MDCT) and magnetic resonance imaging (MRI) in the evaluation of the mandibular invasion by squamous cell carcinomas (SCC) of the oral cavity. Correlation with pathological data. J Exp Clin Cancer Res 2010;29:73.

13. Gu DH, Yoon DY, Park CH, et al. CT, MR, (18)F-FDG PET/CT, and their combined use for the assessment of mandibular invasion by squamous cell carcinoma of the oral cavity. Acta Radiol 2010;51:1111–9.

14. Imaizumi A, Yoshino N, Yamada I, et al. A potential pitfall of MR imaging for assessing mandibular invasion of squamous cell carcinoma in the oral cavity. AJNR Am J Neuroradiol 2006;27(1):114–22.

15. Sturgis EM, Wei Q, Spitz MR. Descriptive epidemiology and risk factors for head and neck cancer. Semin Oncol 2004;31(6):726–33.

16. Bhattacharyya N, Nayak VK. Survival outcomes for second primary head and neck cancer: a matched analysis. Otolaryngol Head Neck Surg 2005; 132(1):63–8.

17. Petersson F. Nasopharyngeal carcinoma: a review. Semin Diagn Pathol 2015;32(1):54–73.

18. Glastonbury CM, Salzman KL. Pitfalls in the staging of cancer of nasopharyngeal carcinoma. Neuroimaging Clin N Am 2013;23(1):9–25.

19. Liao XB, Mao YP, Liu LZ, et al. How does magnetic resonance imaging influence staging according to AJCC staging system for nasopharyngeal carcinoma compared with computed tomography? Int J Radiat Oncol Biol Phys 2008;72(5):1368–77.

20. Vokes EE, Liebowitz DN, Weichselbaum RR. Nasopharyngeal carcinoma. Lancet 1997;350(9084): 1087–91.

21. Trotta BM, Pease CS, Rasamny JJ, et al. Oral cavity and oropharyngeal squamous cell cancer: key imaging findings for staging and treatment planning. Radiographics 2011;31(2):339–54.

22. Chaturvedi AK, Engels EA, Pfeiffer RM, et al. Human papillomavirus and rising oropharyngeal cancer incidence in the United States. J Clin Oncol 2011; 29(32):4294–301.

23. Hsu WC, Loevner LA, Karpati R, et al. Accuracy of magnetic resonance imaging in predicting absence of fixation of head and neck cancer to the prevertebral space. Head Neck 2005;27(2):95–100.

24. Kuno H, Onaya H, Fujii S, et al. Primary staging of laryngeal and hypopharyngeal cancer: CT, MR imaging and dual-energy CT. Eur J Radiol 2014; 83(1):e23–5.

25. Becker M, Zbaeren P, Delavelle J, et al. Neoplastic invasion of laryngeal cartilage: reassessment of criteria for diagnosis at CT. Radiology 1997;203(2): 521–32.

26. Becker M, Zbaeren P, Casselman JW, et al. Neoplastic invasion of laryngeal cartilage: reassessment of criteria for diagnosis at MR imaging. Radiology 2008;249(2):551–9.

27. Kuno H, Onaya H, Iwata R, et al. Evaluation of cartilage invasion by laryngeal and hypopharyngeal squamous cell carcinoma with dual-energy CT. Radiology 2012;265(2):488–96.

28. Beitler JJ, Muller S, Grist WJ, et al. Prognostic accuracy of computed tomography findings for patients with laryngeal cancer undergoing laryngectomy. J Clin Oncol 2010;28(14):2318–22.

29. Szewczyk-Bieda MJ, White RD, Budak MJ, et al. A whiff of trouble: tumours of the nasal cavity and their mimics. Clin Radiol 2014;69(5):519–28.

30. Som PM, Shapiro MD, Biller HF, et al. Sinonasal tumors and inflammatory tissues: differentiation with MR imaging. Radiology 1988;167(3):803–8.

31. Som PM, Brandwein-Gensler MS, Kassel EE, et al. Tumors and tumor-like conditions of the sinonasal cavities. In: Som PM, Curtin HD, editors. Head and neck imaging. 5th edition. St Louis (MO): Mosby; 2011. p. 1912.

32. Kontzialis M, Glastonbury CM, Aygun N. Evaluation: imaging studies. Adv Otorhinolaryngol 2016;78: 25–38.

33. Friedman ER, Saindane AM. Pitfalls in the staging of cancer of the major salivary gland neoplasms. Neuroimaging Clin N Am 2013;23(1):107–22.

34. Christe A, Waldherr C, Hallett R, et al. MR imaging of parotid tumors: typical lesion characteristics in MR imaging improve discrimination between benign and malignant disease. AJNR Am J Neuroradiol 2011;32(7):1202–7.

35. Moonis G, Cunnane MB, Emerick K, et al. Patterns of perineural tumor spread in head and neck cancer. Magn Reson Imaging Clin N Am 2012;20(3):435–46.

36. Matsusue E, Fujihara Y, Matsuda E, et al. Differentiating parotid tumors by quantitative signal intensity evaluation on MR imaging. Clin Imaging 2017;46: 37–43.

37. Freling N, Crippa F, Maroldi R. Staging and follow-up of high-grade malignant salivary gland tumours: The role of traditional versus functional imaging approaches - a review. Oral Oncol 2016;60:157–66.

38. Bui CD, Ching AS, Carlos RC, et al. Diagnostic accuracy of 2-[fluorine-18]fluro-2-deoxy-D-glucose positron emission tomography imaging in nonsquamous tumors of the head and neck. Invest Radiol 2003;38(9):593–601.

39. Park HL, Yoo Ie R, Lee N, et al. The value of F-18 FDG PET for planning treatment and detecting recurrence in malignant salivary gland tumors: comparison with conventional imaging studies. Nucl Med Mol Imaging 2013;47(4):242–8.

40. Ghantous Y, Naddaf R, Barak M, et al. The role of fine needle aspiration in the diagnosis of parotid gland tumors: correlation with preoperative computerized tomography tumor size. J Craniofac Surg 2016;27(2):e192–6.

41. Kim HJ, Kim JS. Ultrasound-guided core needle biopsy in salivary glands: a meta-analysis. Laryngoscope 2018;128(1):118–25.

42. Lydiatt WM, Mukherji SK, O'Sullivan B, et al. Major salivary glands. In: AJCC cancer staging manual. 8th edition. New York: Springer; 2017.

43. Maroldi R, Farina D, Borghesi A, et al. Perineural tumor spread. Neuroimaging Clin N Am 2008;18(2): 413–29, xi.

44. Garden AS, Weber RS, Morrison WH, et al. The influence of positive margins and nerve invasion in adenoid cystic carcinoma of the head and neck treated with surgery and radiation. Int J Radiat Oncol Biol Phys 1995;32(3):619–26.

45. Badger D, Aygun N. Imaging of perineural spread in head and neck cancer. Radiol Clin North Am 2017; 55(1):139–49.

46. Lee JR, Kim JS, Roh JL, et al. Detection of occult primary tumors in patients with cervical metastases of unknown primary tumors: comparison of (18)F FDG PET/CT with contrast-enhanced CT or CT/MR imaging-prospective study. Radiology 2015;274(3): 764–71.

47. Kwee TC, Kwee RM. Combined FDG-PET/CT for the detection of unknown primary tumors: systematic review and meta-analysis. Eur Radiol 2009;19(3): 731–44.

48. Sadick M, Schoenberg SO, Hoermann K, et al. Current oncologic concepts and emerging techniques in the diagnosis of oral cancer. GMS Curr Top Otorhinolaryngol Head Neck Surg 2012;11:Doc08.

49. Som P, Brandwein MS. Lymph nodes. In: Som PM, Curtin HD, editors. Head and neck imaging. 5th edition. St Louis (MO): Mosby; 2011. p. 1912.

50. Aiken AH, Poliashenko S, Beitler JJ, et al. Accuracy of preoperative imaging in detecting nodal extracapsular spread in oral cavity squamous cell carcinoma. AJNR Am J Neuroradiol 2015;36(9):1776–81.

51. Roh JL, Park JP, Kim JS, et al. 18F fluorodeoxyglucose PET/CT in head and neck squamous cell carcinoma with negative neck palpation findings: a prospective study. Radiology 2014;271(1):153–61.

52. Brink I, Klenzner T, Krause T, et al. Lymph node staging in extracranial head and neck cancer with FDG PET-appropriate uptake period and size-dependence of the results. Nuklearmedizin 2002; 41(2):108–13.

53. Hyde NC, Prvulovich E, Newman L, et al. A new approach to pre-treatment assessment of the N0 neck in oral squamous cell carcinoma: the role of sentinel node biopsy and positron emission tomography. Oral Oncol 2003;39(4):350–60.

54. Schroeder U, Dietlein M, Wittekindt C, et al. Is there a need for positron emission tomography imaging to stage the N0 neck in T1-T2 squamous cell carcinoma of the oral cavity or oropharynx? Ann Otol Rhinol Laryngol 2008;117(11):854–63.

55. Fleming AJ Jr, Smith SP Jr, Paul CM, et al. Impact of [18F]-2-fluorodeoxyglucose-positron emission tomography/computed tomography on previously untreated head and neck cancer patients. Laryngoscope 2007;117(7):1173–9.

56. Saito N, Nadgir RN, Nakahira M, et al. Posttreatment CT and MR imaging in head and neck cancer: what the radiologist needs to know. Radiographics 2012; 32(5):1261–82.

57. Lobert P, Srinivasan A, Shah GV, et al. Postoperative and postradiation changes on imaging. Otolaryngol Clin North Am 2012;45(6):1405–22.

58. Garcia MR, Passos UL, Ezzedine TA, et al. Postsurgical imaging of the oral cavity and oropharynx: what radiologists need to know. Radiographics 2015;35(3):804–18.

59. Choi SH, Lee JH, Choi YJ, et al. Detection of local tumor recurrence after definitive treatment of head and neck squamous cell carcinoma: histogram analysis of dynamic contrast-enhanced T1-weighted perfusion MRI. AJR Am J Roentgenol 2017;208(1): 42–7.

60. Roman BR, Patel SG, Wang MB, et al. Guideline familiarity predicts variation in self-reported use of routine surveillance PET/CT by physicians who treat head and neck cancer. J Natl Compr Canc Netw 2015;13(1):69–77.

61. Gourin CG, Boyce BJ, Williams HT, et al. Revisiting the role of positron-emission tomography/computed tomography in determining the need for planned neck dissection following chemoradiation for advanced head and neck cancer. Laryngoscope 2009;119(11):2150–5.

62. Pryor DI, Porceddu SV, Scuffham PA, et al. Economic analysis of FDG-PET-guided management of the neck after primary chemoradiotherapy for node-positive head and neck squamous cell carcinoma. Head Neck 2013;35(9):1287–94.

63. Mueller J, Huellner M, Strobel K, et al. The value of (18) F-FDG-PET/CT imaging in oral cavity cancer patients following surgical reconstruction. Laryngoscope 2015;125(8):1861–8.

64. Aiken AH, Farley A, Baugnon KL, et al. Implementation of a novel surveillance template for head and neck cancer: neck imaging reporting and data system (NI-RADS). J Am Coll Radiol 2016; 13(6):743–6.

65. De Felice F, de Vincentiis M, Valentini V, et al. Follow-up program in head and neck cancer. Crit Rev Oncol Hematol 2017;113:151–5.

66. Krieger DA, Hudgins PA, Nayak GK, et al. Initial performance of NI-RADS to predict residual or recurrent head and neck squamous cell carcinoma. AJNR Am J Neuroradiol 2017;38(6):1193–9.

Multidisciplinary Team Planning for Patients with Head and Neck Cancer

Thomas D. Shellenberger, DMD, MD[a],*,
Randal S. Weber, MD[b]

KEYWORDS

- Head and neck cancer • Multidisciplinary care • Tumor board • Quality indicators
- Cancer outcomes • Quality of life • Integrated delivery of health care

KEY POINTS

- The multidisciplinary planning conference is a critical point in the evaluation and management of patients with head and neck cancer in determining outcome and quality of life.
- The management of patients with head and neck cancer is complex and dictates the care of a multidisciplinary team for optimal results.
- The head and neck multidisciplinary team ensures the complete evaluation of patients before beginning treatment.
- The head and neck multidisciplinary team improves the accuracy of diagnosis and staging of patients on which to base the most appropriate treatment.
- The head and neck multidisciplinary team improves the outcomes of treatment by following the best available evidence through clinical practice guidelines and treatment algorithms, and by engaging in clinical research trials.

Quia parvus error in principio magnus est in fine.(A small error at the outset is a large one in the end)
— *St Thomas Aquinas, On Being and Essence[1]*

At no point in the evaluation and management of a patient with cancer are the details so important in determining the outcome of treatment as at that moment when the multidisciplinary team, known as the tumor board, first meets to discuss the case. At the treatment planning conference, team members present comprehensive information about each patient: the pathologic diagnosis, disease stage, performance status, psychosocial conditions, and (perhaps most important of all) the patient's intentions. They seek the expertise of team members across a range of disciplines. They consider evidence-based strategies, evaluate guidelines, and review the inclusion criteria of clinical trials. After careful consideration, they reach a consensus on the goals of treatment. Their effective communication across medical specialties initiates coordinated, continuous care. Owing to the complexity of their care, optimal treatment of patients with head and neck cancer depends on a multidisciplinary team approach. Because even a small error can become a big one, the tumor board is a critical determinant of the outcome of treatment. The consequences of

---

Disclosure: The authors have nothing to disclose.
[a] Division of Surgical Oncology, Banner MD Anderson Cancer Center, 2946 East Banner Gateway Drive, Suite 450, Gilbert, AZ 85234, USA; [b] Department of Head and Neck Surgery, University of Texas MD Anderson Cancer Center, 1515 Holcombe Boulevard, Unit 1445, Houston, TX 77030, USA
* Corresponding author.
E-mail address: Thomas.Shellenberger@bannerhealth.com

Oral Maxillofacial Surg Clin N Am 30 (2018) 435–444
https://doi.org/10.1016/j.coms.2018.06.005
1042-3699/18/© 2018 Elsevier Inc. All rights reserved.

any errors made in diagnosis, staging, or any of the other important factors that determine the outcome of cancer care are magnified along the course of treatment. Given that effective communication is essential to the proper function of the team, only a multidisciplinary team approach can offer the best chances of getting it right from the start.

A well-functioning multidisciplinary team ensures complete assessment of the patient before treatment. The team approach also improves the accuracy of diagnosis and staging on which treatment is based and directs treatment to the identified goals from the outset. The result is a plan of care offering the best chances for cure by adhering to evidence-based approaches and practice guidelines. At the same time, treatment-related morbidity can be reduced by addressing patient function and quality of life. Moreover, the multidisciplinary team brings a unified voice to the treatment plan on behalf of the patient. The team stands united for the purpose of achieving the common goals of oncologic results, preserving or restoring of function, and the relieving suffering. When these goals are discussed at the outset of treatment, the team has the best chance of arriving at a patient-centered, personalized, efficient, and value-driven plan of care. Considering the impact of cancer treatment on daily function and quality of life, its financial burdens, and the disappointing outcomes of secondary treatment of recurrent cancer, the best chance for a favorable outcome is clearly the first chance, with definitive initial therapy.[2]

This article discusses how multidisciplinary teams coordinate the complex care of patients with head and neck cancer. It outlines the rationale for multidisciplinary care with a focus on the specific needs of patients with head and neck cancer and describes how multidisciplinary teams function. It also reviews the research on the impact of multidisciplinary care on diagnostic and staging accuracy, patient outcomes, the management of treatment-related adverse events, adherence to evidence-based guidelines, and recruitment into clinical trials.

THE COMPLEXITY OF CARE

Getting it right from the start begins with a deep appreciation of the complexity of caring for patients with head and neck cancer. That complexity lies in the variety of head and neck cancers, the paucity of level I evidence from randomized trials, the frequent use of multimodal treatment of head and neck cancers, and the diversity of surgical demands. Moreover, the effects of head and neck cancer and its treatment on bodily form and function, and therefore quality of life, add to the unique challenges of this disease. Thus, the complexity of head and neck cancer demands a multidisciplinary approach to meet the goals of individual patients.

Malignancies of the head and neck differ from other cancer types in their heterogeneity and their rarity. The overall incidence and prevalence of head and neck cancers is low in most countries. In 2017, some 63,030 new cases of oral cavity, pharyngeal, and laryngeal cancers were estimated to occur, accounting for about 3.7% of new cancer cases in the United States.[3] Thus, malignancies of the head and neck comprise a small fraction of the whole cancer landscape, especially compared with breast, prostate, lung, and colorectal cancers. Importantly, head and neck cancer is not a single disease but a group of diseases that differ in their site of origin, cause, and histology. The treatment, prognosis, and quality of life of a patient with a T2 cancer of the oral cavity and a patient with a T2 cancer of the larynx can differ dramatically, as can those of patients with oropharyngeal cancers related to human papilloma virus and oropharyngeal cancers related to smoking or those of patients with squamous cell carcinoma and those with mucoepidermoid carcinoma of the base of the tongue. The great burden of morbidity and mortality imposed by head and neck cancer demands the optimal care of patients from the time of diagnosis through the end of life. According to statistics of the National Cancer Database, the overall survival for stage IV cancers of the head and neck remains less than 50% at 5 years.[4]

Clinical trials have improved the treatment of cancers that are more homogeneous and more prevalent than head and neck cancers. The design, execution, and interpretation of high-quality prospective trials by expert panels with multidisciplinary members have led to the development of evidence-based strategies and guidelines that have improved the treatment of many cancer types. However, high-quality evidence from randomized controlled trials of head and neck cancer treatments is lacking because of obstacles in enrolling adequate numbers of patients in centers where trials are available. As a result, treatment decisions for individual patients often rest on the practitioner's experience and skill set, personal bias and philosophy, and the availability of resources at the treatment center.

Unlike patients with most other types of cancer, most patients with head and neck cancers are treated with multiple modalities, including surgery, radiation, conventional chemotherapy, and more recently targeted therapy or immunotherapy. Although a single modality of treatment may be appropriate in patients who present with early-stage disease, 60% to 70% of patients with head and neck cancer present with locally or regionally advanced disease.[5] Combined modality therapy is thus generally recommended for most patients with head and neck cancer. The use of multiple modalities adds greatly to the complexity of care and requires teams of multiple physicians from an array of disciplines and subspecialties. Moreover, with multimodal therapy, patients with head and neck cancer are at an increased risk of treatment-related morbidity.

Surgery for head and neck cancer has the goals of both ablation and reconstruction to offer the best chance of cure while minimizing the impact of surgery on the patient's quality of life. The oncologic goal of surgery is complete microscopic resection of the primary tumor along with the regional lymph node basin at risk for spread. However, the anatomic complexity of the region demands the involvement of surgeons from several disciplines, including neurosurgery and thoracic surgery, and of head and neck surgeons with subspecialties in, for example, skull base surgery or transoral laser surgery. The functional implications of ablative surgery are generally addressed at the time of initial surgery to avoid delays in the administration of adjuvant therapy, optimize rehabilitative efforts, and maximize quality of life. Therefore, the input of plastic and reconstructive surgeons is also critical to developing the treatment plan from the outset. An optimal surgical plan depends on effective discussion of the advantages and disadvantages of various surgical approaches among multiple subspecialists.

Head and neck cancer threatens vital functions, such as speaking, breathing, chewing, and swallowing, as well as facial form and body image. Advanced disease and disease at certain sites can threaten vision or hearing or cause other kinds of neurologic impairment. The disease's effects on facial form and body image carry psychosocial manifestations. Patients in the workforce additionally face the threat of disability that harms their ability to provide for their families. Multidisciplinary teams, therefore, should include rehabilitative specialists, social workers, and mental health professionals. The complexity of care for patients with cancer now demands no less than all a multidisciplinary team has to offer.

Perhaps no factor is more important in the treatment of patients with head and neck cancer than the impact of the disease and of treatment sequelae on patients' quality of life. One of the biggest challenges for head and neck oncologists is helping patients discover for themselves what quality of life means to them and to define the treatment goals that are most important to them. Because quality of life can vary dramatically between individuals and across a single individual's lifetime, discussions of quality of life should begin at the first contact with the patient. However, that discussion should also emphasize that life is always a good, and this is a quality that can never be lost. Because quality is always diminished by disease, the focus should be not on whether a patient's life will have enough quality to it but whether a treatment would be unduly burdensome and insufficiently beneficial for the patient's particular circumstances.[6]

THE FUNCTION OF THE MULTIDISCIPLINARY TEAM

According to the *Clinical Practice Guidelines in Oncology* of the National Comprehensive Cancer Network (NCCN), all patients with head and neck cancer need access to the full range of support services and specialists with expertise in the management of head and neck cancer.[5] Multidisciplinary team care is now widely accepted as a best practice for the treatment of head and neck cancer. Multidisciplinary care has evolved over recent decades from a scarce resource available only in academic centers in major metropolitan areas to the standard of care in cancer treatment and is increasingly being implemented in cancer care services worldwide. Only a multidisciplinary team can meet the complex decision-making demands required for the assessment and treatment of patients with head and neck cancer.

The tumor board is a multidisciplinary group of specialists with experience and expertise in their respective fields, all dedicated to the care of patients with cancer, as discussed in the NCCN Guidelines® for Head and Neck Cancers (https://www.nccn.org/professionals/physician_gls/default.aspx#head-and-neck). Multidisciplinary disease management can be delivered through multidisciplinary clinics, where team members examine the patient, order and perform diagnostic procedures and tests, and discuss treatment options. Then, at the multidisciplinary team planning conference, team members synthesize their findings; discuss diagnosis, staging, and treatment options; and offer a formal recommendation for a plan of care. Planning conferences may be held weekly and are attended by core members of the multidisciplinary team.[7]

For example, at The University of Texas MD Anderson Cancer Center, informal interdisciplinary cooperation among surgeons, radiation oncologists, oncologic dentists, medical oncologists, and speech pathologists evolved into a formal treatment planning conference in the early 1980s. The head and neck service's planning conference was one of the first at MD Anderson and in the nation, and it has endured with minor modifications to the present day. The complexities of multidisciplinary care, with a wide variety of specialists participating in the care of patients with cancer, have demanded the establishment of treatment algorithms and decision support tools.[8] Over the last few decades, multidisciplinary care has increasingly been implemented in cancer care services in many countries, with up to 80% of patients undergoing care by a multidisciplinary team in some locations.[7]

However, discussion by the multidisciplinary team focused on advocating for the patient should not be limited to the time of initial diagnosis and treatment planning. A dynamic multidisciplinary team planning conference should also be fluid enough to accommodate needs that arise in managing complications during treatment, assessing response to disease, monitoring for recurrence after treatment, and even attending to late effects of treatment. Follow-up should be performed by physicians and other health care professionals with expertise in the management and prevention of treatment sequelae.[5] Patients can greatly benefit from active discussion among their team throughout course of disease.[9]

More than 100 years ago, William J. Mayo, who launched the first multispecialty clinic, argued that "it [has become] necessary to develop medicine as a co-operative science; the clinician, the specialist, and the laboratory workers united for the good of the patient."[10] The growing knowledge of molecular and cellular biology and immunology, advances in surgical and functional rehabilitation, and the ongoing challenges of treating cancer have made medicine more complex than ever before. Clinicians' response to these challenges must be equally strong. The first priority is ensuring the complete evaluation of the patient by all members of the multidisciplinary team.

ENSURING COMPLETE EVALUATION

The multidisciplinary team helps get it right from the start by ensuring that patients' evaluations are complete before they embark on treatment. By presenting the available data and interpreting the findings of physical, endoscopic, pathologic, and imaging examinations, the members of the multidisciplinary team can determine the optimal extent of evaluation for individual patients. For instance, they can determine whether biopsy specimens are adequate or whether additional

testing is needed, or they can assess whether additional or complementary imaging studies are required. Perhaps most importantly, members of the multidisciplinary team, ancillary support staff, or other consultants can be enlisted if their input is critical to developing a tailored approach for each patient.

A study by Kelly and colleagues[11] provided evidence that tumor board meetings ensure a complete evaluation of patients with head and neck cancer. When patients were treated by a multidisciplinary team, adherence to clinical quality indicators improved compared with the era before a multidisciplinary team was instituted at the same center. For example, the rate of dental evaluation increased by more than 2-fold and the rate of nutritional assessment increased by nearly 2-fold after a formal head and neck tumor board was introduced. These more complete evaluations before treatment initiation enable proactive management and enhance communication with the goal of minimizing morbidity during treatment.

Evaluation of speech and swallowing and counseling for cessation of smoking and alcohol consumption are important parts of a comprehensive evaluation and should be considered benchmarks in pretreatment evaluation. Shellenberger and colleagues[12] found the reproducibility of established guidelines for pretreatment evaluation in a cohort of patients with head and neck cancer treated by a multidisciplinary team. Several factors in the pretreatment evaluation were measured as data end points in the medical record to objectively assess the completeness of evaluation. By establishing benchmarks, teams can review their practice patterns to guide program development and ensure adherence to quality standards.

Efficiency of Care

The complete evaluation of the patient by the multidisciplinary team also sets the stage for efficient care. A timely and complete evaluation of patients with head and neck cancer can prevent delays in treatment that can compromise treatment results, frustrate trial enrollment, and cause patients to be dissatisfied with their care. A report on the adoption of a multidisciplinary team approach for patients with head and neck cancer in a United States Veterans Administration hospital system found that both access to and timeliness of care were improved. Significant improvements were found in the time to first visit after initial consult and the time from biopsy to the initiation of treatment. The adoption of the multidisciplinary team also increased the number of pretreatment consultations referred to providers outside of the core team by 4-fold.[13] Townsend and colleagues[14] compared a cohort of patients with newly diagnosed head and neck cancers evaluated in a multi-appointment traditional clinic with those evaluated in a single-day multidisciplinary clinic. Patients evaluated in the single-day multidisciplinary clinic with a built-in tumor board discussion experienced significantly fewer instances of delay greater than 30 days from referral to initiation of treatment than did those evaluated in the traditional clinic. Considering that longer time to initiation of treatment has been correlated with shorter overall survival in patients with squamous cell carcinoma of the head and neck,[15] the cost of delays in treatment can be great. Similarly, Rosenthal and colleagues[16] showed that, for patients with a total treatment package time of less than 100 days, rates of locoregional disease control and survival at 2 years were significantly higher than for those with a package time of more than 100 days. Delays in care thus affect the timing of adjuvant therapy to the detriment of outcomes. Delays in initiating radiation treatment as a result of prolonged postoperative hospitalization, undue dental evaluation or extractions, obstacles in the placement of percutaneous endoscopic gastrostomy tubes, or unplanned breaks in radiation all have the potential to increase treatment package time and compromise the chance of cure.

The findings of Murphy and colleagues[17] underscored how frequently patients experience treatment delays; their study of a National Cancer Database cohort of more than 50,000 patients undergoing curative-intent therapy found that 1 in 4 patients met with a delay in treatment. In 2011, the most recent year of the study for which data are available, 25% of patients waited more than 46 days from initial diagnosis to the initiation of curative treatment. Delays in treatment were independently correlated with adverse outcomes: the risk of death was higher in patients who waited more than 46 days than in those who waited for less than 30 days. Therefore, even highly efficient multidisciplinary teams should strive to coordinate treatment planning in the most expeditious manner possible.

Managing Comorbidities

Patients with head and neck cancer present a unique blend of characteristics. They often have comorbidities such as cardiac and pulmonary disease, which have some risk factors in common with head and neck cancer. Weber and colleagues[18] reported on the impact of medical comorbidities on important measures of quality after operations for head and neck cancer. In a cohort of 2618 surgical patients, 47% had significant cardiovascular disease, 12% had diabetes, and 6% had chronic obstructive pulmonary disease. More than half of the patients had some type of comorbidity, and 17% had 2 or more comorbidities. Patients undergoing higher-acuity surgical procedures were nearly twice as likely to have multiple comorbidities and twice as likely to have a postoperative course complicated by 2 or more negative surgical performance factors. A thorough evaluation for medical optimization and risk stratification by an expert member of the multidisciplinary team is critical to understanding the impact of patients' comorbidities on their cancer care.

Social and Psychological Care

Many patients newly diagnosed with cancer are beset by a host of personal and family stressors that must be considered in the overall scheme of care. Patients also have values that require careful consideration and discussion in the context of their care. The extent to which psychosocial and family support are available can have dramatic impact on the treatment goals, treatment selection, and the prospects of success. What quality of life means can vary dramatically among patients, their spouses and family members, and even at various points along an individual patient's continuum of care.

A cancer navigation program can ensure the completeness of the evaluation by the multidisciplinary team and promote the continuity and uniformity of care. As a key member of the multidisciplinary team, a navigator can prevent patient dissatisfaction with service fragmentation, delays in access, lack of information, and lack of coordination between providers. As cancer care options have become increasingly complex, patients and families must balance multiple cancer-related demands. They often complain about a sense of isolation, feelings of powerlessness, and a lack of guidance about whom to reach and where to go when they need information about their disease, treatment, and side effects. Fillion and colleagues[19] reported on a cancer navigation model for patients with head and neck cancer that improved continuity of care; enhanced patient satisfaction; reduced the duration of hospitalizations; empowered patients to cope with cancer-related problems, including body image concerns; and improved patients' emotional quality of life. Oncology nurses performing navigation can play an important role not only in ensuring continuity of care but also in providing supportive care; helping patients to cope better with cancer treatments, recovery, cancer progression, and end-of-life issues.

Ultimately, the duty of the planning conference is not merely to provide a recommendation based on the tumor characteristics but instead to deeply consider the whole patient; to listen carefully to patients' priorities; and to recommend a treatment plan that can best meet the goals established by the patient, rather than goals that might be imposed on the patient. Educating patients to make well-informed decisions will most likely result in a treatment plan that is the most meaningful to patients and their families.

IMPROVING THE ACCURACY OF DIAGNOSIS AND STAGING

Another way in which the multidisciplinary team helps get it right from the start is by improving the accuracy of diagnosis and staging. The appropriate treatment can only be selected by accurate diagnosis and staging. The results of the comprehensive examination of the head and neck[5] are considered by the team members. By carefully reviewing the available pathologic specimens and imaging studies, the team arrives at an accurate diagnosis. Accurate staging also depends on critical review of a host of factors by all members of the team to reach consensus.

Diagnosis

Before the meeting of the tumor board, the diagnosis is based mainly on the report of a biopsy performed and interpreted before the referral of the patient to the treating physician. This report is generally from a community pathologist, whose experience with and expertise in the subtleties and nuances of head and neck pathology may be highly variable. A review of the available biopsy slides with the multidisciplinary team's pathologist can bring subspecialty-level expertise to bear on the findings. Establishing the diagnosis may depend on specific objective criteria or may require additional testing, such as staining with immunohistochemistry for biomarkers. The presence or absence of pathologic factors such as perineural invasion and extracapsular spread can greatly affect decision making. Moreover, input from other members of the team can offer insight into the context of the findings, such as the site of the biopsy, the effects of prior treatment, and the relation to imaging findings. As a result, both the diagnosis and the status of important pathologic factors can be revised during the discussion of the tumor board, resulting in a more accurate foundation on which to base treatment decisions.

Because establishing the correct diagnosis on which to base appropriate treatment is so critical to the outcome, pathologists with subspecialty expertise are essential members of the multidisciplinary team. The value of conducting a second review of pathologic specimens is underscored by the findings of a comprehensive study of the diagnostic error rate among patients with cancer treated at a tertiary care hospital before initiation of treatment. Middleton and colleagues[20] found differences between the original pathology report and the subspecialty final pathology report in up to 25% of cases. Among head and neck pathology reports, the rate of discordance was even higher, with differences between original and final pathology reports in 46% of cases. Although some of these discrepancies were considered minor, up to one-third resulted in a change in the diagnosis that affected patient care.

The impact of multidisciplinary team meetings on patient assessment and diagnosis was evaluated in a systematic review of the literature by Pillay and colleagues.[21] In 27 studies, changes in assessment and diagnosis following multidisciplinary team meetings were found in up to 45% of patients. In addition to changes in pathologic interpretation, review of radiologic imaging at the multidisciplinary team meeting changed the diagnosis in 10% of cases in one of the studies included in the review.[22]

Changes in the diagnosis and staging of patients presented at the head and neck multidisciplinary planning conference can have a profound effect on the recommendation for treatment, especially in cases of high-grade, advanced-stage tumors. Wheless and colleagues[23] quantified the impact of the multidisciplinary tumor board discussion on the treatment of patients with head and neck cancer. In a prospective cohort of 120 patients with head and neck tumors, 27% of patients whose cases were presented for discussion had some change in tumor diagnosis, stage, or treatment plan from the preconference plan. Moreover, these changes most frequently resulted in escalation in management by the addition of multimodal care.

The extent to which diagnosis and staging changes occur when cases are discussed by multidisciplinary teams was underscored in a retrospective analysis by Bergamini and colleagues.[24] The investigators found a need for additional investigation in 50% of patients with head and neck cancer evaluated at a tertiary referral center and changes in diagnosis, staging, or treatment plan in more than 60% of these patients. The investigators pointed out that nonspecialists referred patients to the multidisciplinary team for access to new investigations and treatment modifications specific to patients with rare types of head and neck cancer. Bergamini and colleagues also suggested that evaluation by a multidisciplinary team has the benefit of reduced health care costs, because it optimizes therapy and minimizes adverse events.

Staging

The disease stage at diagnosis is the most important factor in predicting survival rates and guiding treatment in patients with head and neck cancer. Accurate staging is also critical to informing patients and their families about the prognosis and the possibility of cure with available treatment options. Moreover, with accurate staging, the goals of treatment can be defined in relation to treatment-associated morbidities and their impact on the patient's quality of life. The staging of cancer requires a complex integration of objective data to arrive at an accurate determination of the extent of disease at diagnosis. Critical factors determining the staging of head and neck cancers include the subsite and size of the primary tumor; invasion of the cortical bone, inferior alveolar nerve, floor of the mouth, or skin of the face; invasion of adjacent structures, such as the deep muscles of the tongue or maxillary sinus; and involvement of the masticatory space, pterygoid plates, skull base, or internal carotid artery. Because it is the most important prognostic factor for oral cavity cancer, the status of the lymph node basin at risk should be determined with the utmost accuracy. The number and size of metastatic lesions and the side of the neck involved should be ascertained by clinical examination and Imaging and aided by cytology in selected cases before treatment. The presence of distant metastasis should be ascertained by the most accurate means available, because the finding of distant metastasis shifts treatment priorities away from locoregional to systemic treatment. Each of the elements of staging requires careful consideration. Accurate staging is determined by interpreting the findings of clinical and endoscopic examinations, conventional and specialized imaging, and pathologic reports. Therefore, expert input is required of each member of the multidisciplinary team.

Evidence suggests that multidisciplinary teams improve the accuracy of staging at diagnosis for patients with head and neck cancer and that this improvement likely translates into improved outcomes. In a study of patients included in an Australian tumor registry, Friedland and colleagues[25] found a higher likelihood of advanced disease in patients treated by a multidisciplinary team than in those treated with a different approach. Nonetheless, patients with stage IV disease treated by the multidisciplinary team had better survival rates than did similarly staged patients treated outside of a multidisciplinary setting, suggesting that multimodality therapy and advances in chemotherapy made available through multidisciplinary care benefitted those patients.

IMPROVING THE OUTCOMES OF TREATMENT

By getting it right from the start, the multidisciplinary team affords patients the best chance for cure with the least impact on quality of life. By carefully interpreting the data from a complete evaluation and by establishing an accurate diagnosis and stage, the goals of treatment can be clearly defined. The best among the available treatment options can be selected: the treatment that offers the greatest likelihood of benefit and the least likelihood of harm. The extent to which evidence-based strategies can be applied to individual cases can be determined by the team members who best understand the strengths and limitations of the available evidence. National or institutional guidelines for care can be considered to determine the extent to which individual patients are within or outside such frameworks. In addition, individual patients can be considered for the research trials that are most likely to benefit both their own care and the goals of the study. Therefore, care can be delivered with the best value and highest quality at the lowest cost.

The impact of multidisciplinary planning on outcomes in patients with head and neck cancer can be difficult to evaluate in prospective studies. Outcomes are improved when patients with head and neck cancers are treated in high-volume centers.[5] Wuthrick and colleagues[26] reported a nearly 2-fold increased risk of death (hazard ratio = 1.91) and decreased 5-year overall survival rate (from 69.1% to 51.0%) among patients treated in Radiation Therapy Oncology Group trials at historically low-accruing centers (1–12 patients over the 5-year period) compared with patients treated at historically high-accruing centers (>41 patients). However, the extent to which the multidisciplinary team approach contributed to this difference is not clear. Although studies have shown improved disease-free and overall survival in patients treated with multimodal therapy, of which multidisciplinary planning is a part,[27,28] none have shown improvements in outcomes that can be solely attributed to the multidisciplinary planning conference. A prospective trial in which patients are randomized to an arm in which their treatment is not planned by the multidisciplinary team could not be justified. Nonetheless, the impact of multidisciplinary team planning on outcomes can be inferred from factors strongly associated with outcomes, including adherence to evidence-based strategies in care and clinical practice guidelines and enrollment of patients in clinical trials.

Evidence-Based Care

The multidisciplinary team uses the available evidence to determine the diagnostic and treatment interventions that are most likely to offer benefit and least likely to do harm. Whether a center follows the best available evidence supported by multidisciplinary teams and endorsed by expert panels also offers insight into the quality of care it delivers. The multidisciplinary team planning conference thus ensures that the individualized cancer treatment plan is tailored to the tumor site and stage, the patient's comorbidities, and the patient's goals and desires.

By eliciting the input of physicians with subspecialty expertise in the management of head and neck cancer (those who are best able to critically interpret the results of clinical trials), the multidisciplinary planning conference grounds its treatment approach in evidence-based medicine. The selection of an evidence-based treatment approach tends to decrease the variation in practice patterns, both within the multidisciplinary team and between centers, while better ensuring the judicious use of limited health care resources. High-quality evidence provides a rationale for specific recommendations and offers a source of education for medical professionals, patients, and families. When care is provided in accordance with high-quality evidence, treatment outcomes improve and resource use often decreases, along with the cost of care.[7]

Appealing to the available high-quality evidence provides an important set of checks and balances that prevents any dominant personality or specialty within a given multidisciplinary team from imposing a personal preference or bias on the decision-making process. A well-documented, evidence-based plan that may be referred to on an ongoing basis can facilitate the coordination of care, because the expectations of treatment are defined at the outset. Evidence-based approaches further aid in identifying the usual options of care that define a standard. As El Saghir and colleagues[7] point out, occasional deviation by a multidisciplinary team from the recommendations of high-quality evidence is expected and is likely to reflect high-quality cancer care; usual deviation by a multidisciplinary team from the recommendations of high-quality evidence is very likely to reflect biased, poor-quality cancer care.[7]

Applying high-quality evidence requires commitment from the multidisciplinary team and from the supporting infrastructure of the center in which the care is delivered. Resources, systems, and expertise are required to follow evidence-based guidelines. Modifying recommendations that are based on high-quality evidence can be justified only in practice environments in which resources are so limited that evidence-based treatment cannot be provided.

Clinical Practice Guidelines and Cancer Treatment Algorithms

The multidisciplinary team planning conference ensures that treatment options are uniformly recommended among patients evaluated by the team and that these options rest on an established standard, such as the guidelines published by the NCCN[5] (www.nccn.org) or the treatment algorithms published by The University of Texas MD Anderson Cancer Center[29] (https://www.mdanderson.org/for-physicians/clinical-tools-resources/clinical-practice-algorithms/cancer-treatment-algorithms.html). Cancer treatment algorithms depict best practices for care delivery and describe a multidisciplinary approach for evaluation, diagnosis, treatment, and surveillance of various malignancies. These algorithms were developed by multidisciplinary panels that interpreted the best available evidence and offered their experience and expert recommendations. Although no patients fit precisely into guidelines or algorithms, these tools are valuable because they help to avoid treatments that are likely to be ineffective or even harmful. Thus, the guidelines should be adjusted for individual patients as circumstances dictate. The use of guidelines and algorithms by a multidisciplinary team with a clear understanding of their strengths and limitations can improve overall care.

Adherence to clinical practice guidelines may also serve as a measure of the quality of care delivered for types of cancer for which process-specific and outcome-specific validated metrics are lacking. The extent to which a multidisciplinary team's recommendations and treatment comply with clinical practice guidelines is thus likely to influence the value of the care as well as disease-free and overall survival. A retrospective review by Lewis and colleagues[30] found that multidisciplinary teams' recommendations (86.6% of the time) and actual treatment (86.3% of the time) usually complied with NCCN guidelines. Among a cohort of 232 patients with previously untreated incident cancers of the head and neck, a significant overall survival benefit was found for patients who underwent the treatment recommended by the multidisciplinary team (hazard ratio = 0.49; 95%

confidence interval = 0.27–0.89; P = .02). Thus, assessing the congruence between the multidisciplinary team's recommendation and the actual treatment offers great insight into the uniformity of care. Moreover, assessing predictors of noncompliance with guidelines can help identify trends and center-specific practice patterns that affect care. Such insight can lead the multidisciplinary team to modify its approaches or to justify alternative strategies.

Nonetheless, achieving optimal treatment outcomes for patients with head and neck cancer requires more than simply following established guidelines. Studies have shown that following guidelines outside of a multidisciplinary team context does not achieve adequate outcomes. Sharma and colleagues[31] showed that Medicare patients with advanced-stage head and neck cancer at high-volume hospitals not specifically complying with NCCN recommendations had better survival outcomes than did patients treated at low-volume hospitals that were practicing NCCN-compliant care plans. These findings suggest that the function of the multidisciplinary team is a critical determinant of outcomes and that adherence to guidelines outside the setting of a multidisciplinary team can fall short in achieving the goals of care.

Guidelines and algorithms are best applied to patients who are part of the population for which the algorithms were developed. Recommendations should never be followed at the expense of the sound clinical judgment of physicians. Guidelines should be considered for all patients and tailored to individual patients in whom important differences are present.

Clinical Research

Even as changes in the delivery of cancer care abound, overall survival for patients with head and neck cancer has changed little over the last several decades. A host of questions are yet to be answered in hopes of optimizing treatment outcomes. Every multidisciplinary team thus owes its patients the debt of learning from the experience of every patient under its care. The new knowledge needed to advance the field emerges from clinical research trials designed to answer a broad range of questions, carefully designed by members of the multidisciplinary team, and incorporated into strategies that can be shared between institutions. In the head and neck tumor board, the cases of individual patients are considered with regard to the research questions they pose. Inclusion criteria, performance status, and other patient factors can be reviewed to determine whether a patient fits into an available trial. Patients whose cases are discussed at a head and neck tumor board that includes a research coordinator are more likely to be enrolled in clinical trials. In addition, patients for whom standard therapy has failed can be considered for a range of available options tailored to them or referred to another center where they can get the best trial option.

SUMMARY: MAKE IT MATTER MOST FROM THE START

Getting it right from the start serves patients by offering the best chances to be cured of their disease with the lowest cost in terms of morbidity. It is an honor and privilege to care for patients with head and neck cancer, and the multidisciplinary team owes a great debt to each patient undergoing treatment. Because not every patient presenting to the multidisciplinary team can be assured of a curative outcome, preserving every patient's quality of life is the team's paramount goal. Efforts to expand the possibilities of oncologic treatment options with the likelihood of success should always be tempered against the ethical concerns that care is beneficial, useful, and not burdensome for individual patients to fully respect their human dignity. No matter the prognosis, the team can always provide compassionate care and alleviate suffering. No individual provider or specialist can meet all the needs of every individual patient, but an integrated multidisciplinary team can offer the best chances of achieving treatment goals. The team members must strive to know their patients well from the beginning in order to establish the goals most relevant to the patient and to offer the best chances of achieving those goals. Multidisciplinary teams leave a legacy to patients with head and neck cancer by advancing the field through the knowledge and insight gained by treating their patients. By constantly aiming to improve care, by increasing the comparability of data across institutions, by forming networks between sites through clinical trials, and by building national cancer treatment paradigms, multidisciplinary teams make the treatment of every patient matter most.

REFERENCES

1. Aquinas T. Prologue. In: On being and essence. Pontifical Institute on Mediaeval Studies; 1968. p. 1. Translated by Armand Maurer.
2. Goodwin WJ Jr. Salvage surgery for patients with recurrent squamous cell carcinoma of the upper aerodigestive tract: when do the ends justify the means? Laryngoscope 2000;110(3 Pt 2 Suppl 93):1–18.
3. Siegal RL, Miller KD, Jemal A. Cancer statistics, 2017. CA Cancer J Clin 2017;67:7–30.

4. National cancer database. Available at: https://www. facs.org/quality-programs/cancer/ncdb, Accessed March 20, 2018.

5. NCCN clinical practice guidelines in oncology (NCCN guidelines). Head and neck cancers. Version 2. 2018. Available at: https://www.nccn.org/ professionals/physician_gls/default.aspx#head-and-neck. Accessed August 6, 2018.

6. A Catholic Guide to End-of-Life Decisions, The National Catholic Bioethics Center1998; rev. 2005; rev.2011.

7. El Saghir NS, Keating NL, Carlson RW, et al. Tumor boards: optimizing the structure and improving efficiency of multidisciplinary management of patients with cancer worldwide. Am Soc Clin Oncol Educ Book 2014;e461–6. https://doi.org/10.14694/ EdBook_AM.2014.34.e461.

8. Goepfert H. History and evolution. In: The University of Texas MD Anderson Cancer Center Department of Head and Neck Surgery Our History. Houston (TX): MD Anderson Media Services; 2015. p. 1–3.

9. Heineman T, St John MA, Wein RO, et al. It takes a village: the importance of multidisciplinary care. Otolaryngol Clin North Am 2017;50(4):679–87.

10. Olson JS, Lee Clark R. History, and the dread disease. In: Making cancer history. Baltimore (MD): The Johns Hopkins University Press; 2009. p. 20.

11. Kelly SL, Jackson JE, Hickey BE, et al. Multidisciplinary clinic care improves adherence to best practice in head and neck cancer. Am J Otolaryngol 2013;34(1):57–60.

12. Shellenberger TD, Tseng J, Manon R, et al. Concordance with established guidelines by the multidisciplinary team in the management of patients with head and neck cancer. abstract of the Global Academic Programs. Oslo (Norway): 2012.

13. Patil RD, Meinzen-Derr JK, Hendricks BL, et al. Improving access and timeliness of care for veterans with head and neck squamous cell carcinoma: a multidisciplinary team's approach. Laryngoscope 2016;126(3):627–31.

14. Townsend M, Kallogjeri D, Scott-Wittenborn N, et al. Multidisciplinary clinic management of head and neck cancer. JAMA Otolaryngol Head Neck Surg 2017;143(12):1213–9.

15. van Harten MC, Hoebers FJ, Kross KW, et al. Determinants of treatment waiting times for head and neck cancer in the Netherlands and their relation to survival. Oral Oncol 2015;51(3):272–8.

16. Rosenthal DI, Liu L, Lee JH, et al. Importance of the treatment package time in surgery and postoperative radiation therapy for squamous carcinoma of the head and neck. Head Neck 2002;24(2):115–26.

17. Murphy CT, Galloway TJ, Handorf EA, et al. Survival impact of increasing time to treatment initiation for patients with head and neck cancer in the United States. J Clin Oncol 2016;34(2):169–78.

18. Weber RS, Lewis CM, Eastman SD, et al. Quality and performance indicators in an academic department of head and neck surgery. Arch Otolaryngol Head Neck Surg 2010;136(12):1212–8.

19. Fillion L, de Serres M, Cook S, et al. Professional patient navigation in head and neck cancer. Semin Oncol Nurs 2009;25(3):212–21.

20. Middleton LP, Feeley TW, Albright HW, et al. Second-opinion pathologic review is a patient safety mechanism that helps reduce error and decrease waste. J Oncol Pract 2014;10(4):275–80.

21. Pillay B, Wootten AC, Crowe H, et al. The impact of multidisciplinary team meetings on patient assessment, management and outcomes in oncology settings: a systematic review of the literature. Cancer Treat Rev 2016;42:56–72.

22. Greer HO, Frederick PJ, Falls NM, et al. Impact of a weekly multidisciplinary tumor board conference on the management of women with gynecologic malignancies. Int J Gynecol Cancer 2010;20(8):1321–5.

23. Wheless SA, McKinney KA, Zanation AM. A prospective study of the clinical impact of a multidisciplinary head and neck tumor board. Otolaryngol Head Neck Surg 2010;143(5):650–4.

24. Bergamini C, Locati L, Bossi P, et al. Does a multidisciplinary team approach in a tertiary referral centre impact on the initial management of head and neck cancer? Oral Oncol 2016;54:54–7.

25. Friedland PL, Bozic B, Dewar J, et al. Impact of multidisciplinary team management in head and neck cancer patients. Br J Cancer 2011;104(8):1246–8.

26. Wuthrick EJ, Zhang Q, Machtay M, et al. Institutional clinical trial accrual volume and survival of patients with head and neck cancer. J Clin Oncol 2015; 33(2):156–64.

27. Liao CT, Kang CJ, Lee LY, et al. Association between multidisciplinary team care approach and survival rates in patients with oral cavity squamous cell carcinoma. Head Neck 2016;38(Suppl 1):E1544–53.

28. Wang YH, Kung PT, Tsai WC, et al. Effects of multidisciplinary care on the survival of patients with oral cavity cancer in Taiwan. Oral Oncol 2012; 48(9):803–10.

29. Cancer treatment algorithms. Oral cavity cancer. Available at: www.mdanderson.org/for-physicians/ clinical-tools-resources/clinical-practice-algorithms/ cancer-treatment-algorithms.html. Accessed February 28, 2018.

30. Lewis CM, Nurgalieva Z, Sturgis EM, et al. Improving patient outcomes through multidisciplinary treatment planning conference. Head Neck 2016; 38(Suppl 1):E1820–5.

31. Sharma A, Schwartz SM, Méndez E. Hospital volume is associated with survival but not multimodality therapy in Medicare patients with advanced head and neck cancer. Cancer 2013;119(10): 1845–52.

Oral Assessment and Management of the Patient with Head and Neck Cancer

Herve Y. Sroussi, DMD, PhD[a],*, Maryam Jessri, DDS, PhD[b],
Joel Epstein, DMD, MSD, FRCD(C), FDS RCS(Edin)[c]

KEYWORDS

- Head and neck cancer • Oral cavity • Oral health • Quality of life

KEY POINTS

- Patients undergoing treatment of head and neck cancer (HNC) risk developing significant acute and chronic changes of the oral cavity and the head and neck region.
- Understanding the cause and pathophysiology to predict and manage the course of these changes can improve the impact on survivorship.
- Although treatment approaches for HNC are evolving rapidly, peer-reviewed evidence in the prevention, identification, and management of their sequalae is currently limited.
- Current understanding is limited to case reviews and anecdotal clinical experience.

INTRODUCTION

Patients undergoing treatment of head and neck cancer (HNC) risk developing significant acute and chronic changes of the oral cavity and the head and neck region. The treatment modalities of surgery, radiation therapy (RT), and chemotherapy, alone or in combination, result in significant acute and chronic changes of the oral cavity. These alterations are not limited to the hard tissue (teeth and alveolar bone) and oral mucous membrane, but also affect the soft tissues of the head and neck. The consequences of cancer treatment can significantly impair the quality of life of patients with HNC. Therefore, understanding the cause and pathophysiology to predict and manage the course of these changes can improve the impact on survivorship.

The role of oral health providers in the management of patients with HNC covers a wide variety of services from the time of diagnosis through survivorship.[1] This article offers considerations and recommendations for patients before, during, and after treatment of HNC to maintain oral health, compensate for treatment consequences, and improve quality of life. Although treatment approaches for HNC are evolving rapidly, peer-reviewed evidence in the prevention, identification, and management of their sequalae is currently limited. Newly approved immunotherapeutic approaches in the treatment of HNC, although promising oncologically, may further complicate the course of treatment. Current understanding is limited to case reviews and anecdotal clinical experience. Here, we present evidence-based recommendations and expert opinion.

Disclosure: The authors have nothing to disclose.
[a] Division of Oral Medicine and Dentistry, Brigham and Women's Hospital, Dana-Farber Cancer Institute, 1620 Tremont Street, Suite BC-3-028H, Boston, MA 02120, USA; [b] Division of Oral Medicine and Dentistry, Brigham and Women's Hospital, 1620 Tremont Street, Suite BC-3-028H, Boston, MA 02120, USA; [c] Division of Otolaryngology and Head and Neck Surgery, City of Hope, 1500 East Duarte Road, Duarte, CA 91010, USA
* Corresponding author.
E-mail address: hsroussi@bwh.harvard.edu

ASSESSMENT AND MANAGEMENT BEFORE CANCER TREATMENT

Evaluation of the oral cavity in patients before treatment of HNC aims to determine immediate dental and mucosal needs while especially considering complications that might be anticipated with cancer treatment. Although not all oral complications of cancer treatment can be prevented, their timely recognition, diagnosis, and appropriate management can significantly improve the quality of life in survivors of HNC. An important consideration is the historically increased incidence of HNC in socioeconomically deprived populations and the unfortunately associated greater risk of dental infections in these patients.[2,3] Acute odontogenic infection during cytotoxic chemotherapy can potentially threaten life. In addition, periapical and periodontal infections, and dental extractions, may predispose patients to developing osteoradionecrosis (ORN) of the jaw after RT.[4,5]

Although a comprehensive oral assessment and management should be completed before cancer treatment, the time required to complete that management must be carefully considered to avoid a potential delay in beginning cancer treatment that might impact the overall survival. A retrospective analysis of the National Cancer Database for the interval from the time of diagnosis to the time of beginning curative treatment, defined as the time to treatment initiation (TTI), in patients with HNC showed a median of 20 to 28 days for HNC stage I through IV.[6] Several studies have reported a significant increase in the risk of death in patients with delayed TTI compared with those with faster access to curative treatment.[6–8] Murphy and colleagues[6] reported that a TTI equal or greater than 91 days increased the risk of overall mortality of patients with HNC by 23% (95% confidence interval, 15%–32%) when compared with people with a TTI equal to or less than 30 days.

Saliva at Baseline

Saliva has essential functions in maintaining oral health, which are classified into overlapping categories: (1) lubrication, (2) protective, (3) wound healing, (4) taste and smell and (5) digestion, and (6) tooth remineralization.[9] Salivary flow has been estimated to range from 0.3 to 0.4 mL/min at rest and 1 to 2 mL/min on stimulation.[10] In a state of salivary hypofunction, which is generally defined as resting flow of less than 0.1 mL/min, salivary functions are compromised.

Individuals may be at increased risk of developing dry mouth before receiving treatment of HNC. HNC has a greater incidence in older patients, in whom dry mouth is a common side effect of polypharmacy.[11] A few examples of medications that may cause hyposalivation include anticholinergic drugs (tricyclic antidepressants, antipsychotics, antihistamines, and anticholinergic drugs for overactive bladder), sympathomimetic drugs (antidepressants, appetite depressants, and β_2-agonist bronchodilators), antihypertensive medications, cytotoxic drugs, opioid and benzodiazepines, and antimigraine agents.[11] Underlying systemic diseases, such as Sjögren syndrome, diabetes mellitus, rheumatoid arthritis, and hypothyroidism, have also been independently associated with hyposalivation.[11] Although some authors have shown clearly impaired function of salivary glands in older patients, others attribute these findings to the confounding effects of medications.[12–14] Although saliva is composed mostly of water (99%), the quality and composition of the saliva are also essential contributors to oral health.[15]

Although only a small number of patients with HNC (6%) reported dry mouth before treatment, decrease in the amount of saliva during and after treatment in patients with pre-existing dry mouth justifies evaluation of salivary flow before cancer treatment.[16] In addition, given the individual differences, measuring stimulated and unstimulated saliva before initiation of treatment of HNC provides a better understanding of patient's baseline and helps tailor the best possible care for each patient.[16] As a whole, it is recommended that a pretreatment baseline evaluation of the stimulated and unstimulated salivary flow be conducted to better document this morbidity and offer an intervention based on objective measurement of dysfunction.

Temporomandibular Joint Health and Mouth Opening at Baseline

Temporomandibular joint function is affected as a late effect of RT.[17] Secondary to radiation, the masseter, temporalis, and pterygoid muscles can experience inflammatory changes that can lead to muscle fibrosis. The effect of RT on muscle function may be compounded with postsurgical scarring and result in limited mouth opening (trismus) with a potentially progressive course.[18]

Trismus impacts activities of daily living, such as eating, speaking, or performing routine oral homecare. Trismus can also become a barrier to accessing regular professional dental care. These complications may result in rapid deterioration of oral health with profound consequences on the quality of life of cancer survivors.

Accordingly, baseline measurement of mouth opening and continued monitoring is recommended for patients with HNC. Progressive loss of mouth opening is addressed proactively through physical therapy and exercise. The establishment of baseline clinical data is crucial to early recognition of developing trismus.

Dental

The two most prominent goals of stabilizing the oral cavity to maintain good oral health in patients with HNC are preventing oral infection during RT and chemotherapy and avoiding the need for dentoalveolar surgery after RT.

Caries (restorable vs unrestorable)

The loss of equilibrium between demineralization and remineralization of tooth structure eventually results in cavitation defined as dental caries. A highly complex process with several key components, saliva plays an important role in preventing caries by balancing the pH, by cleansing and antimicrobial effects, and by providing the source for mineralizing teeth.[19] Patients with HNC from socioeconomically deprived populations also lack access to dental prevention and care resulting in a higher risk of dental caries.[20]

The natural history of dental caries begins as the reversible demineralization of enamel progressing to irreversible cavitation of tooth structure, ultimately requiring invasive treatment and leading to pain, the spread of infection to jaw bones, and the progression to extraction of the tooth. In patients with HNC who have undergone RT, dental extractions increase the risk of developing ORN. Therefore, a comprehensive oral examination with appropriate dental radiographs is recommended to evaluate the baseline dental status and to devise a treatment plan.[21] At this stage, teeth with restorable caries should be identified and addressed. Because the mandibular molar region is a high-risk area for developing ORN, attentive treatment of these teeth before RT followed by close monitoring and management after RT is recommended.[5]

To achieve a short TTI, teeth with a hopeless prognosis that require extraction should be prioritized to provide the patient with as much time as possible between dental extraction and beginning RT. Although the aim is to complete all dental procedures before the initiation of curative cancer treatment, limited time may dictate that treatment of teeth with excellent prognosis or with superficial caries is completed during or early after curative cancer treatment.

Pulpal health and root canal therapy evaluation

To ensure that all acute and chronic sources of intraoral infection and soft tissue trauma are managed before initiation of RT, patients should undergo clinical examination and obtain dental radiographs. Teeth with evidence of endodontic infection, such as periapical radiolucency in a nonvital tooth, abnormal or nonresponsive pulp-test, and deep caries extending to the pulp chamber, are recommended for root canal therapy (RCT) before beginning RT if deemed restorable. Similarly, teeth with large restorations, with suspicious carious lesions, or with sensitivity should be evaluated for vitality and treated with endodontic therapy if necessary before beginning RT. It should be remembered that in some cases, definitive treatment may mean extraction.

For teeth with periapical radiolucency and prior RCT, old radiographs should be compared whenever possible to differentiate scarring from failed endodontic treatment. Symptomatic teeth with a history of prior endodontic treatment should be re-evaluated and treated if necessary by repeating endodontic therapy or extraction before RT.

It is noteworthy that effective cleaning of the root canal and coronal seal of RCT-treated teeth are important components of treatment success, whereas the lack of an effective coronal seal results in treatment failure.[22]

Root tips

If possible, all retained root tips should be extracted before RT. Alternatively, appropriate cases are managed by RCT and submerging the root fragment. Bony impacted root tips without evidence of periapical pathology and that have shown stability over a long period of time can be monitored rather than extracted.

Third molars

Partially erupted third molars with infection, those with previous history of pericoronitis, or teeth whose management is likely to complicate cancer treatment should be removed before RT.[23,24] However, removal of third molars is associated with postextraction complications in patients with cancer. The need for prompt TTI further complicates decision making in pretreatment dental management.[23] Therefore, a generalized recommendation for removal of third molars is impractical. Each case should be evaluated individually with final decisions based on patient age, complexity of removal of the third molar, TTI, and the likelihood of complications following cancer therapy if the tooth is retained.

Periodontal Health, Tooth Mobility, and Prognosis

Periodontitis is a common inflammatory and microbial disease that may result in pain, acute infection, and tooth loss. Because poor periodontal health has been associated with ORN, periodontal evaluation and treatment is an integral aspect of screening before RT[25] and of maintenance after cancer therapy. A retrospective analysis of 185 patients with HNC showed that those with inadequately treated periodontal disease (defined as presence of pockets ≥ 6 mm) were more likely to develop severe oral sequelae including ORN.[26]

Additional complications faced by patients with pre-existing periodontal disease, including hyposalivation, shift in microbiota, and rapid loss of tooth-supporting tissues, increase the risk of developing ORN in patients with HNC who undergo RT.[27]

Teeth with severe periodontal involvement, those with grade greater than or equal to two mobility, and teeth with advanced attachment loss of pocketing are recommended for extraction before RT.[28,29] In noncompliant patients who would not commit to diligent self-cleaning and professional cleaning of teeth with furcation involvement and in patients with teeth in the high dose volume or RT, extraction is also indicated.[28] Furthermore, patients should be educated on the importance of commitment to life-long maintenance for improving their periodontal health.

Patient Education

Becoming familiar with the treatment modalities aimed at cancer and the effects expected on oral health is crucial from ethical and practical standpoints. Patients should understand the anticipated morbidities of treatment in the short and long term. Appreciating the prognosis of oral morbidities is important to patients because several of may be long lasting or even permanent. The recommended behavioral modifications including an intensified homecare protocol and more frequent professional visits should be discussed early and at every opportunity.

Patient education should be incorporated early in management, ideally at the pretreatment oral evaluation. Discussing with the patient the rationale for the evaluation and for the recommended treatment approach, especially dental extractions, is vital. In patients with advanced dental or periodontal disease who have had infrequent access to professional oral care and who will undergo RT, education is even more important. Discussing the rationale for recommending dental extractions presents an opportunity to explain the risks of ORN and the recommendation for life-long preventative home care in hopes of preventing the future needs for extractions following RT. Patients should be explained the expected morbidities during treatment, such as mucositis or dysgeusia, and long-term complications, especially hyposalivation and trismus along with their associated risks of dental caries, periodontal diseases, and opportunistic mucosal fungal infections. Patient education provides opportunities to reinforce oral care, such as oral hygiene and fluoride use, diet instruction, and cessation of tobacco and alcohol.

Oral Hygiene

The effectiveness of oral hygiene should be evaluated and encouraged at every opportunity. If mouth pain from oral mucositis prevents homecare, relief may be established with topical anaesthetics, such as viscous lidocaine, before brushing or flossing. The Multinational Association of Supportive Care in Cancer has published fact sheets that can be distributed to patients as educational tools. These resources are available at http://www.mascc.org/patient-education.

Dental Demineralization Prevention

Fluoride supplements, bland mouth rinses, avoiding high-sugar food and drinks between meals, and good oral hygiene are essential components of oral care instructions for patients to minimize the risks of dental demineralization. Toothpaste with 1.1% sodium fluoride (Prevident 5000 plus, Colgate-Palmolive, New York, NY) together with a calcium phosphate preparation supports remineralization of teeth. Additionally, the use of mouth wash containing fluoride is introduced as part of the routine homecare instructions. Mouthwash should be free of alcohol and mild in taste so that use is not discouraged when mucosal pain and sensitivity are expected during and often early after cancer treatment. Oral homecare instructions should be taught, demonstrated, evaluated, and reinforced at every visit.

Modification of the Diet

Addressing diet is an important aspect in the management of patients with HNC. Excessive weight loss must be avoided during and after cancer treatment. The diet of patients may be affected by mouth and throat pain, dental pain, dysgeusia, and odynophagia, or further complicated by hyposalivation and xerostomia.

Chemotherapy and RT to the oral cavity can affect all aspects of taste. The taste for sweet, sour, bitter, salt, and umami (savory test) are all affected but to different degrees. Umami may decrease with therapy, as the other basic tastes, although recovery may be delayed and loss may be permanent. Because umami taste is an important inducer of appetite, the loss can impair intake and threaten the weight stability of patients with HNC.[30]

Dietary counseling should be considered in patients with HNC. Simple strategies of increasing spice, if tolerated, and increasing umami flavoring is suggested. During the worst period of acute mucositis when mucosal pain and odynophagia are most severe, a soft and blend diet is required. Dietary supplements should be recommended and tube feeding may be necessary in cases of severe mucositis.[31] Oral health providers should understand the dietary challenges and provide guidance for patients.[32]

ASSESSMENT AND MANAGEMENT DURING AND AFTER CANCER TREATMENT

Survivors of HNC face challenges that affect oral function and quality of life including taste changes, mucosal sensitivity, hyposalivation, oral infection, increased risk of dental disease, fibrosis and trismus, tissue necrosis, and lymphedema. Oral symptoms demand the attention of oncologists and dental professionals to facilitate diagnosis and appropriate treatment, and to promote patient compliance with treatment recommendations.

Patients after treatment of HNC should be monitored closely to reinforce prevention, early diagnosis, and management of late complications. Optimal oral care is critical to prevent these complications because patients may underreport oral complications. Timely identification of local recurrence and metastasis leading to early referral is paramount for patients treated for upper aerodigestive cancers at high risk.[33,34] Prompt recognition and diagnosis is required for effective management of oral infection; residual mucositis; sensory changes, such as mucosal sensitivity and pain, taste changes; altered salivation; dental and periodontal disease; soft tissue and bone necrosis; and temporomandibular joint disorders.[35] Follow-up dental visits should be tailored to individual patient conditions, although at least twice yearly (**Table 1**).

Patients should be instructed on daily atraumatic tooth brushing and interdental cleaning,[36,37] bland oral rinses if dry mouth continues, and prevention of dental demineralization. Ultrasonic or electric brushes may be recommended, although soft or supersoft manual toothbrushes may be effective.[38] Prescription fluoride is recommended for dentate patients and supplemented by calcium in patients with severe dry mouth to support mineralization of the teeth.

Rich carbohydrates from dietary sources or supplements to support energy intake, and medications sweetened with sucrose, should be avoided if possible or taken with meals after which oral hygiene is best performed.[4]

Mucositis

Mucositis is a symptomatic, dose-limiting toxicity of cytotoxic chemotherapy for HNC that affects virtually all patients undergoing treatment. Signs and symptoms typically develop after the second week of RT and may continue for weeks to months, particularly in patients treated with concurrent chemotherapy.[39] The World Health Organization has published one of the scales used to measure and document oral mucositis (**Table 2**). It is important to assess and document the mucositis grade to better provide supportive care during and after treatment.

Oral mucositis initially presents as erythema of the oral mucosa within the first 1 to 2 weeks of RT and peaks near the end of RT to form pseudomembranous ulcers that may last up to 1 to 2 months after RT.[40] Occasionally, mucositis may become chronic and persist for an extended period of time after RT. Although there is no standard definition for chronic mucositis, the term implies "oral mucosal lesion, that is, atrophy, swelling, erythema, and/or ulceration (as in the immediate acute type of mucositis) which developed or remained at least 3 months post-therapy, after other etiologies have been ruled out."[41]

The anatomic distribution of oral mucositis is generally reflective of the radiation dose; nevertheless, nonkeratinized mucosa is more commonly affected.[42] Patients treated with concurrent chemoradiation and particularly those treated with epidermal growth factor inhibitors are more likely to experience severe mucositis.[42–44] Ulceration and pain are the two main morbidities of oral mucositis that adversely affect the quality of life of patients with HNC and increase the cost of care.[39,45]

Chronic mucosal sensitivity may be more likely to occur in patients who experience severe, acute mucosal damage during treatment and can persist indefinitely after treatment, adversely affecting quality of life. Management includes frequent use of bland oral rinses of saline and bicarbonate, stimulation of saliva whenever possible, and palliative use of agents forming a film or coating. Additionally, lubricating mucosal-coating agents and topical analgesics or anesthetics may be used as needed. Mouthwashes containing alcohol or phenol, having low pH, or flavored with mint may be intolerable. Foods with acidic or spicy qualities, and coarse or abrasive texture may also be challenging for patients.[46,47] Thorough and consistent oral hygiene is needed.

Currently, consensus recommendations for the management of oral mucositis in patients with HNC are generally directed at symptomatic management with topical and systemic analgesics and the use of coating agents.[48,49] Topical anesthetics, such as lidocaine, benzocaine, and diphenhydramine mixed with Maalox (Novartis, Basel, Switzerland), with or without an antifungal

Table 1
Oral care pre– and post–cancer treatment in head and neck cancer survivors

Pre–cancer treatment	• Pretreatment assessment 2–3 wk before cancer therapy • Comprehensive head and neck, oral mucosa, dental, and periodontal examination • Radiographs to assess dental and periodontal status • Baseline jaw range of motion (interincisal opening), baseline resting, and stimulated saliva • Advanced caries, advanced periodontal disease: definitive treatment may require surgery with goal of 1–2 wk of healing time • Periodontal debridement maintenance; oral hygiene instruction • Custom fluoride carriers, custom oral positioning devices

During cancer treatment	• Individual treatment as cancer type and planned treatment indications
	• Oral hygiene reinforced
	• Small carious lesions may be treated with fluoride and/or sealants; daily fluoride applications
	• Symptom management: for pain use topical analgesic and anesthetic agents, systemic analgesics; for dry mouth use hydration, oral rinses and coating agents, lip management
	• Mucositis reduction: patient education
	  ○ Regular brushing, flossing; prosthesis cleaning
	  ○ Bland oral rinses, water based/wax or lanolin lip lubricant
	  ○ Fluoridated toothpaste; or home fluoride trays daily in high-risk patients
	  ○ Soft toothbrushes; electric or ultrasonic brushes for tolerated patients
	  ○ Supersoft brush for severe mucositis or foam brush with chlorhexidine if brushing not possible
	  ○ Dietary instruction; nutritional guidance, tobacco and alcohol avoidance

Post–cancer treatment	• Monitoring, prevention, and management of oral complications (mucositis, dry mouth, mucosal pain, taste change, infection, dental demineralization, dental caries, periodontal disease, soft tissue/osteonecrosis, and so forth)
	• Checking for cancer recurrence or secondary primary cancer
	• Dental caries prevention, periodontal maintenance
	• Determine frequency of dental hygiene follow-up interval based on level of hyposalivation, demineralization/caries rate, and patient's oral hygiene postradiotherapy; patients with dry mouth may require hygiene and recall every 3–4 mo
	• Patient education
	  ○ Fluoridated toothpaste; in high-risk patients home fluoride trays daily
	  ○ Good oral hygiene, soft toothbrushes or electric or ultrasonic brushes, flossing
	  ○ Maintain lubrication of mouth and lips
	  ○ Encourage noncariogenic diet and cessation of tobacco and alcohol

Table 2
The World Health Organization oral mucositis scale

Grade	Description
0 (none)	None
I (mild)	Oral soreness, erythema
II (moderate)	Oral erythema, ulcers, solid diet is tolerated
III (severe)	Oral ulcers, only liquid diet is possible
IV (life-threatening)	Oral alimentation is impossible

Adapted from WHO. WHO handbook for reporting results of cancer treatment. Geneva (Switzerland): WHO; 1979; with permission.

agent, such as nystatin, comprise a topical rinse commonly referred to as Magic Mouthwash. Magic Mouthwash provides pain relief for up to 30 minutes, but may induce burning, stinging, and taste impairment in contact with ulcerated mucosa.[50] Other topical measures for pain management include topical doxepin and morphine mouthwash, which may provide up to 6 to 8 hours of pain relief.[42,51] Topical coating agents, such as Caphosol (EUSA Pharma, Langhorne, PA), and systemic chemoprotective medications are also used in the management of oral mucositis,[52,53] although data are presently limited to support their use in clinical guidelines. Benzylamine has been recommended for radiation mucositis and topical doxepin and morphine have been suggested for use in mucosal pain.

Importantly, pain caused by mucositis is related to inflammation from tissue damage leading to a nociceptive response and to neuropathic sensitization leading to a neuropathic response, which may be treated with neurologically active medications, such as gabapentin and doxepin.[54–56]

RadOnc Toolbox is a publication of the Multinational Association of Supportive Care in Cancer and the International Society of Oral Oncology that is downloaded as an application or accessed online at https://rotoolbox.com.

Soft Tissue Fibrosis

Fibrosis is a common late effect of RT involving the oral mucosa, the neck, and the temporomandibular joints of the radiated field. RT-induced trismus is a debilitating condition that results from inflammation and subsequent fibrosis in masticatory muscles, particularly the lateral pterygoid muscles. Trismus is defined as mouth-opening less than 35 mm. In a systematic review of the literature, the prevalence ranges from 5% for patients treated with intensity-modulated RT (IMRT) up to 31% for those treated with a combination of chemotherapy and three-dimensional conventional RT.[57]

In addition to trismus, fibrosis of muscles of the tongue and constrictor muscles of the pharynx can impair speech and swallowing. Radiation damage to the neck, which may be compounded by surgery, results in fibrosis leading to limitation in range of movement and in damage to the lymphatic system leading to lymphedema.[58]

Although trismus is a well-documented consequence of RT of the head and neck, little data are available to guide preventative measures and management options.[57,59] Treatment with pentoxifylline and vitamin E, the use of devices to provide active mouth opening, and administration of low-level light therapy are among management options, although none with proven efficacy.[57,60]

Dry Mouth and Thick Saliva

Salivary dysfunction can be classified into three categories: (1) hyposalivation, which is objective reduction of salivary flow; (2) xerostomia, which is subjective sensation of reduced saliva with or without hyposalivation; and (3) alterations of salivary composition.[61] In patients with HNC, xerostomia is a common side effect of RT and can affect up to 93% of the patients during treatment and up to 85.3% of patients after treatment.[16] Resolution or improvement of symptoms of xerostomia may be caused by recovery of salivary gland tissue or accommodation by patients with persistent to dry mouth. With the recent emerging use of IMRT over conventional RT, the incidence of severe xerostomia in long-term follow-up is significantly reduced.[62]

In addition to a decreased quantity of saliva, patients with HNC treated with RT also develop an increased viscosity of saliva. Diagnosis is made by subjective report, clinical examination, and objective measurement of salivary flow. Production of thick saliva after RT is partly explained by the more resilient recovery from the damaging effects of RT to the mainly mucous-secreting major salivary glands compared with serous-secreting glands.[16,63] Thick, mucinous saliva fails to provide adequate lubrication and protection, accumulating in the throat to ineffectively dissolve and distribute tastants and leading to altered sensory perception.

Infections

Patient evaluation is critical in the diagnosis of viral, bacterial, and fungal infections. Diagnosis is challenging during the period of mucositis because signs and symptoms of inflammation and infection may overlap. In patients with neutropenia, the signs and symptoms of infection may be muted by suppression of the inflammatory response adding to the challenges in recognition and diagnosis. Viral infections, such as herpes simplex virus and other herpes viruses, commonly occur in patients treated with chemotherapy, whereas reactivation of chronic herpes simplex virus infection is uncommon in patients with HNC treated with radiation. Acyclovir and valacyclovir are effective in the prevention and treatment of herpes simplex virus.[64,65] In patients with cancer, the oral manifestations of viral infection may be more severe, with an altered presentation involving keratinized and nonkeratinized mucosa, and having a more protracted course. Herpes zoster reactivation is also uncommon.

Bacterial infection caused by dental or periodontal infection may exacerbate. Local therapy with or without antibiotics may be needed. If indicated, antibiotics should be initiated on an empiric basis and tailored once culture data become available for patients failing to respond to treatment. In patients with cancer, obtaining bacterial culture and sensitivity tests is prudent because of potential shifts in oral colonization.[4]

The clinical presentation of oropharyngeal candidiasis may be variable and thus difficult to recognize in the face of mucositis, presenting as white patches, red patches, or as hyperplastic candidiasis, with or without angular cheilitis.[66] Other symptoms, such as coated sensation in the mouth, burning sensation, and altered taste, are associated with candidiasis.

Antifungal topical therapy for local disease is preferred initially, whereas systemic therapy may be reserved for patients in whom topical therapy proves ineffective. A topical agent without sucrose should be chosen particularly in patients with dry mouth.[67,68] Because other fungal species with resistance to antifungal agents are prevalent in patients with cancer, fungal cultures to identify the causative species may be important in guiding therapy, particularly in patients failing to respond.[66] Underlying dry mouth should be recognized and treated with sialagogues to stimulate saliva production, enhance treatment effect, and reduce the risk of recurrence of infection.

Dental Caries

Although radiation can independently affect the mechanical and structural properties of teeth, salivary dysfunction is the main cause of the increased risk of caries in patients with HNC.[69] The process of widespread areas of porous enamel with crater formation and exposure of underlying dentine in the setting of rapid progression has been referred to as "radiation caries." Radiation caries has a sudden onset, is not limited to classic tooth surfaces, has a higher risk of treatment failure, and progresses at a faster rate compared with routine dental caries. In addition to the usual caries-prone sites of the teeth, namely occlusal surfaces and interproximal areas, radiation caries may also primarily affect smooth surfaces and incisal edges and may encircle the cervical aspects of teeth.[70] Active carious lesions are identified clinically 3 months after RT and may result in excessive damage to the dentition 1 year after RT in survivors of HNC.[71]

Review of literature between 2001 and 2008 estimated the overall weighted prevalence of dental caries in HNC survivors at 28.1%.[19] The risk of developing dental caries is higher in patients who have received high-dose radiation to parotid glands.[72] A mean dose of less than 26 Gy to at least one parotid gland increases the likelihood of complete recovery of salivary flow to pretreatment rate.[73] Parotid and possibly submandibular gland-sparing irradiation by using IMRT improves the potential for recovery of salivary flow and decreases the risk of developing rampant dental caries.

The American Cancer Society Head and Neck Cancer Survivorship Care Guidelines recommend that survivors of HNC seek regular professional dental follow-up, close monitoring of oral health, and immediate treatment of dental caries.[74,75] Patients are advised to continue diligent home oral care through brushing; dental flossing; and the use of high fluoride gels, toothpastes, or mouthwashes.

Routine dental follow-up, at least twice annually, promotes early detection and timely management of dental demineralization and caries. In patients with severely reduced salivary flow, poor oral hygiene, rampant caries, or periodontal disease, a more frequent follow-up regimen is recommended.[23] Notably, the rate of compliance with aggressive fluoride therapy in patients decreases with time; the rate of compliance with fluoride gel at 2 years after treatment has been reported at 12%.[76,77] Therefore, compliance should be reinforced at all follow-up medical and dental visits.[78]

Rinsing with chlorhexidine, 0.12%, has been shown to significantly decrease plaque index and salivary *Streptococcus mutans* in patients undergoing head and neck RT.[79,80] Rinsing with chlorhexidine, 0.2%, twice daily was also shown to improve gingival index without altering periodontal pathogens in hematopoietic stem cells transplantation recipients.[81]

Because of the increased risk of dental demineralization, the increase in the number of cariogenic organisms in the oral flora, the shift to a softer more cariogenic diet, and the difficulty in maintaining and accessing oral care, prevention and prompt management of dental caries is essential in maintaining oral health.[82] Although not considered an optimal restorative material in the healthy population, glass ionomer cement may provide better protection against secondary caries in patients with xerostomia and those with history of RT to head and neck. However, glass ionomer cements are prone to losing structural integrity with exposure to fluoride gel, thus close monitoring is recommended.[71]

Osteoradionecrosis

ORN of the jaws is an uncommon, yet severe complication of RT of head and neck that is, defined "as an area of exposed devitalized irradiated bone that fails to heal over a period of 3 to 6 months in the absence of local neoplastic disease."[83] ORN more commonly affects the mandible and can develop spontaneously or secondary to trauma from dental extraction, endodontic or periodontal infections, or from denture-induced trauma.[83,84] ORN may result in pain, recurrent infections, disability, and jaw fractures that adversely affect the quality of life of patients.[84,85]

A systematic review of the literature estimated an overall incidence of ORN at 7%,[83] decreasing to 5% in the era of IMRT. The median time from the initiation of RT to the onset of ORN has been reported to range from 2 to 122 months with most cases developing after dental extraction.[86]

Unlike medication-related osteonecrosis of the jaws, there is no consensus on a staging system and classification for ORN and a variety of criteria, such as clinical presentation, symptoms, radiographic findings, anatomic extension, and even response to hyperbaric oxygen therapy, have been recommended for classification of the disease.[84]

ORN is more frequently associated with doses greater than 60 Gy (at 2 Gy/fraction equivalent) and concurrent chemoradiation therapy. Radiation field size, photon energy, brachytherapy, and fractionation are among other documented radiation-related risk factors. The use of IMRT is anticipated to reduce the incidence and prevalence of ORN.[28]

Because of the strong association of dental extraction after RT with the development of ORN, dental evaluation and removal of teeth in the high-dose RT volume, those with guarded or poor prognosis, and those with significant dental disease before initiation of RT is of great importance.[84] A recent review of the literature did not find the use of hyperbaric oxygen therapy to significantly prevent the development of ORN after dental extractions in radiated patients.[87] Based on institutional experience, Sultan and colleagues[87] recommended atraumatic dental extractions, defined as avoidance of raising gingival flaps and reducing alveolar bone when possible, curettage and irrigation of the extraction socket, and re-evaluation after 2 weeks. Systemic treatment with appropriate antibiotic was recommended with topical chlorhexidine, 0.12%, on the day of dental extraction and continued until healing has occurred.[87]

Early ORN is generally managed with conservative approach through monitoring or sequestrectomy, whereas advanced disease usually requires surgical management.[84] Several medications have been suggested for management of ORN. Tocopherol, or vitamin E, is a free radical scavenger with tumor necrosis factor-α inhibitory effects that has shown promising results in treatment of ORN when combined with another tumor necrosis factor-α inhibitor, pentoxifylline and possibly clodronate.[88,89] Clodronate is unique among the bisphosphonates, acting on the osteoblasts to increase bone formation and reducing fibrosis. In addition, the use of low-level laser to promote wound healing has been reported in a limited case series as a potential additional approach in management.[90] Surgical management may be needed in progressive cases.

Sensory Changes

Taste

Taste and smell perception can also be impaired by RT and chemotherapy in patients treated for HNC.

A systematic review of the literature for determining the prevalence of dysgeusia in patients with HNC showed a weighted prevalence of 66.5% in patients that were treated with RT alone and 76% in patients with RT and chemotherapy.[91]

The appreciation of flavor is a combination of taste and smell functions. Smell alterations may go unnoticed because they can be gradual or may be perceived as taste changes.[92,93] According to a recent systematic review of literature, the prevalence of self-reported post-treatment olfactory dysfunctions was between 30% and 60%. Smell disturbances have been reported at 2 weeks after RT in those who received 20 Gy or more to the olfactory epithelium. In one study, 60% of patients reported the presence of unusual smell with the first dose of RT.[94,95] (Ho AS, Kim Tighiouart M, Mita A, et al: Quantitative survival impact of composite treatment delays in HNC. Submitted for publication.)

In addition to the direct effects of RT and chemotherapy on the mucosa, taste disturbances can occur secondary to hyposalivation. There is no known preventative or curative intervention for taste and smell disturbances. A Cochrane review in 2014 found low-quality evidence for effectiveness of zinc supplements in treatment of dysgeusia and no well-documented evidence of protective effects for amifostine.[96–98] Other approaches discussed include the use of megestrol and cannabinoids.

Mucosal pain and sensitivity

Mucosal sensitivity and pain can affect the quality of life of patients directly or by interfering with daily functions, such as eating and speaking, common chronic complaints in survivors of HNC.[99] Ulceration, atrophy, inflammation or neuropathy secondary to neurotoxicity, oxidative stress, inflammation, and complications of ORN can cause pain and sensitivity of the mucosa.[63,100] Mucosal pain and sensitivity may be a direct consequence of oral mucositis related to chemotherapy and RT, and may persist or even begin after resolution of oral mucositis.[27] Currently there is no known preventative measure for RT-induced mucosal pain. The severity of mucositis correlates directly with persistent pain after RT.

Although neuropathic pain in survivors of HNC may be treatment-induced, other causes, such as tumor infiltration and paraneoplastic syndrome, should be ruled out first.[101] Neuropathic pain does not respond well to opioids.[102] Considering the potential side effects of long-term use of opioids, other treatment options are preferred, such as gabapentin, amitriptyline, clonazepam, and duloxetine.[101]

Cancer Surveillance

The low rate of survival for patients with advanced HNC is generally attributed to persistent or recurrent disease and recurrent or second primary tumors identified during routine follow-up in up to 50%.[103,104] These data confirm the importance of close follow-up and monitoring for patients with a history of HNC. According to the National Comprehensive Cancer Network, survivors of HNC should be followed every 1 to 3 months during the first year after treatment, every 2 to 4 months during the second year, every 4 to 6 months during the third through fifth years, and annually afterward.[105] Compliance with post-treatment surveillance was shown to significantly improve patients' overall survival.[105] The frequency, utility, and imaging schedule following cancer treatment remains under assessment.[106]

SUMMARY

Improvements in therapy and changes in the epidemiology of patients with HNC have led to increasing numbers of survivors and the greater need for continuing management of oral and dental health in this population. Patients with HNC have complex oral health needs, often requiring multidisciplinary collaboration between oncologists and dental professionals with special knowledge in the oral care of patients with cancer. The management of patients with HNC must include evaluation and treatment or supportive care before, during, and after the initiation of therapy.

REFERENCES

1. Epstein JB, Guneri P, Barasch A. Appropriate and necessary oral care for people with cancer: guidance to obtain the right oral and dental care at the right time. Support Care Cancer 2014;22(7): 1981–8.
2. Conway DI, McMahon AD, Smith K, et al. Components of socioeconomic risk associated with head and neck cancer: a population-based case-control study in Scotland. Br J Oral Maxillofac Surg 2010; 48(1):11–7.
3. Johnson S, McDonald JT, Corsten M, et al. Socioeconomic status and head and neck cancer incidence in Canada: a case-control study. Oral Oncol 2010;46(3):200–3.
4. Hong CH, Napenas JJ, Hodgson BD, et al. A systematic review of dental disease in patients undergoing cancer therapy. Support Care Cancer 2010;18(8):1007–21.
5. Kojima Y, Yanamoto S, Umeda M, et al. Relationship between dental status and development of osteoradionecrosis of the jaw: a multicenter retrospective study. Oral Surg Oral Med Oral Pathol Oral Radiol 2017;124(2):139–45.
6. Murphy CT, Galloway TJ, Handorf EA, et al. Survival impact of increasing time to treatment initiation for patients with head and neck cancer in the United States. J Clin Oncol 2016;34(2):169–78.
7. Dahlke S, Steinmann D, Christiansen H, et al. Impact of time factors on outcome in patients with head and neck cancer treated with definitive radio(chemo)therapy. In Vivo 2017;31(5):949–55.
8. van Harten MC, Hoebers FJ, Kross KW, et al. Determinants of treatment waiting times for head and neck cancer in the Netherlands and their relation to survival. Oral Oncol 2015;51(3):272–8.
9. Dawes C, Pedersen AM, Villa A, et al. The functions of human saliva: a review sponsored by the world workshop on oral medicine VI. Arch Oral Biol 2015;60(6):863–74.
10. Proctor GB. The physiology of salivary secretion. Periodontol 2000 2016;70(1):11–25.
11. Saleh J, Figueiredo MA, Cherubini K, et al. Salivary hypofunction: an update on aetiology, diagnosis and therapeutics. Arch Oral Biol 2015;60(2):242–55.
12. Pedersen W, Schubert M, Izutsu K, et al. Age-dependent decreases in human submandibular gland flow rates as measured under resting and post-stimulation conditions. J Dent Res 1985; 64(5):822–5.
13. Shetty SR, Bhowmick S, Castelino R, et al. Drug induced xerostomia in elderly individuals: an institutional study. Contemp Clin Dent 2012;3(2):173–5.
14. Smith CH, Boland B, Daureeawoo Y, et al. Effect of aging on stimulated salivary flow in adults. J Am Geriatr Soc 2013;61(5):805–8.
15. Galvao-Moreira LV, da Cruz MC. Dental demineralization, radiation caries and oral microbiota in patients with head and neck cancer. Oral Oncol 2015;51(12):e89–90.
16. Jensen SB, Pedersen AM, Vissink A, et al. A systematic review of salivary gland hypofunction and xerostomia induced by cancer therapies: prevalence, severity and impact on quality of life. Support Care Cancer 2010;18(8):1039–60.
17. Goldstein M, Maxymiw WG, Cummings BJ, et al. The effects of antitumor irradiation on mandibular opening and mobility: a prospective study of 58 patients. Oral Surg Oral Med Oral Pathol Oral Radiol Endod 1999;88:365–73.
18. Jeremic G, Venkatesan V, Hallock A, et al. Trismus following treatment of head and neck cancer. J Otolaryngol Head Neck Surg 2011;40:323–9.
19. Michelet M. Caries and periodontal disease in cancer survivors. Evid Based Dent 2012;13(3):70–3.
20. Costa SM, Martins CC, Bonfim Mde L, et al. A systematic review of socioeconomic indicators and dental caries in adults. Int J Environ Res Public Health 2012;9(10):3540–74.

21. Devi S, Singh N. Dental care during and after radio-therapy in head and neck cancer. Natl J Maxillofac Surg 2014;5(2):117–25.

22. Eliyas S, Jalili J, Martin N. Restoration of the root canal treated tooth. Br Dent J 2015;218(2):53–62.

23. Hong CHL, Hu S, Haverman T, et al. A systematic review of dental disease management in cancer patients. Support Care Cancer 2017;26(1):155–74.

24. Tai CC, Precious DS, Wood RE. Prophylactic extraction of third molars in cancer patients. Oral Surg Oral Med Oral Pathol 1994;78(2):151–5.

25. Katsura K, Sasai K, Sato K, et al. Relationship between oral health status and development of osteoradionecrosis of the mandible: a retrospective longitudinal study. Oral Surg Oral Med Oral Pathol Oral Radiol Endod 2008;105(6):731–8.

26. Schuurhuis JM, Stokman MA, Roodenburg JL, et al. Efficacy of routine pre-radiation dental screening and dental follow-up in head and neck oncology patients on intermediate and late radiation effects. A retrospective evaluation. Radiother Oncol 2011;101(3):403–9.

27. Sroussi HY, Epstein JB, Bensadoun RJ, et al. Common oral complications of head and neck cancer radiation therapy: mucositis, infections, saliva change, fibrosis, sensory dysfunctions, dental caries, periodontal disease, and osteoradionecrosis. Cancer Med 2017;6(12):2918–31.

28. Duarte VM, Liu YF, Rafizadeh S, et al. Comparison of dental health of patients with head and neck cancer receiving IMRT vs conventional radiation. Otolaryngol Head Neck Surg 2014;150(1):81–6.

29. Duncan GG, Epstein JB, Tu D, et al. Quality of life, mucositis, and xerostomia from radiotherapy for head and neck cancers: a report from the NCIC CTG HN2 randomized trial of an antimicrobial lozenge to prevent mucositis. Head Neck 2005; 27(5):421–8.

30. Yamashita H, Nakagawa K, Hosoi Y, et al. Umami taste dysfunction in patients receiving radiotherapy for head and neck cancer. Oral Oncol 2009;45: e19–23.

31. Epstein JB, Huhmann MB. Dietary and nutritional needs of patients undergoing therapy for head and neck cancer. J Am Dent Assoc 2011;142(10):1163–7.

32. Epstein JB, Huhmann MB. Dietary and nutritional needs of patients after therapy for head and neck cancer. J Am Dent Assoc 2012;143(6):588–92.

33. Kasperts N, Slotman B, Leemans CR, et al. A review on re-irradiation for recurrent and second primary head and neck cancer. Oral Oncol 2005; 41(3):225–43.

34. Kataoka T, Kiyoita N, Shimada T, et al. Randomized trial of standard pain control with or without gabapentin for pain related to radiation-induced mucositis in head and neck cancer. Auris Nasus Larynx 2016;43(6):677–84.

35. Bensinger W, Schubert M, Ang KK, et al. NCCN task force report. Prevention and management of mucositis in cancer care. J Natl Compr Canc Netw 2008;6(Suppl 1):S1–21.

36. Keefe DM, Schubert MM, Elting LS, et al. Updated clinical practice guidelines for the prevention and treatment of mucositis. Cancer 2007;109(5):820–31.

37. Ransier A, Epstein JB, Lunn R, et al. A combined analysis of a toothbrush, foam brush, and a chlorhexidine-soaked foam brush in maintaining oral hygiene. Cancer Nurs 1995;18(5):393–6.

38. Hong CH, daFonseca M. Considerations in the pediatric population with cancer. Dent Clin North Am 2008;52(1):155–81.

39. Elting LS, Cooksley CD, Chambers MS, et al. Risk, outcomes, and costs of radiation-induced oral mucositis among patients with head-and-neck malignancies. Int J Radiat Oncol Biol Phys 2007;68(4): 1110–20.

40. Kostler WJ, Hejna M, Wenzel C, et al. Oral mucositis complicating chemotherapy and/or radiotherapy: options for prevention and treatment. CA Cancer J Clin 2001;51(5):290–315.

41. Elad S, Zadik Y. Chronic oral mucositis after radiotherapy to the head and neck: a new insight. Support Care Cancer 2016;24(11):4825–30.

42. Lalla RV, Saunders DP, Peterson DE. Chemotherapy or radiation-induced oral mucositis. Dent Clin North Am 2014;58(2):341–9.

43. Ang KK, Zhang Q, Rosenthal DI, et al. Randomized phase III trial of concurrent accelerated radiation plus cisplatin with or without cetuximab for stage III to IV head and neck carcinoma: RTOG 0522. J Clin Oncol 2014;32(27):2940–50.

44. Li Y, Chen QY, Tang LQ, et al. Concurrent chemoradiotherapy with or without cetuximab for stage II to IVb nasopharyngeal carcinoma: a case-control study. BMC Cancer 2017;17(1):567.

45. Russo G, Haddad R, Posner M, et al. Radiation treatment breaks and ulcerative mucositis in head and neck cancer. Oncologist 2008;13(8):886–98.

46. Lalla RV, Sonis ST, Peterson D. Management of oral mucositis in patient with cancer. Dent Clin North Am 2008;52(1):61.

47. Sonis ST. Pathobiology of oral mucositis: novel insights and opportunities. J Support Oncol 2007; 5(9 Suppl 4):3–11.

48. Rosenthal DI, Trotti A. Strategies for managing radiation-induced mucositis in head and neck cancer. Semin Radiat Oncol 2009;19(1):29–34.

49. Ruggiero SL, Dodson TB, Fantasia J, et al. American Association of Oral and Maxillofacial Surgeons position paper on medication-related osteonecrosis of the jaw: 2014 update. J Oral Maxillofac Surg 2014;72(10):1938–56.

50. Barasch A, Elad S, Altman A, et al. Antimicrobials, mucosal coating agents, anesthetics, analgesics,

and nutritional supplements for alimentary tract mucositis. Support Care Cancer 2006;14(6):528–32.

51. Sarvizadeh M, Hemati S, Meidani M, et al. Morphine mouthwash for the management of oral mucositis in patients with head and neck cancer. Adv Biomed Res 2015;4:44.

52. Henke M, Alfonsi M, Foa P, et al. Palifermin decreases severe oral mucositis of patients undergoing postoperative radiochemotherapy for head and neck cancer: a randomized, placebo-controlled trial. J Clin Oncol 2011; 29(20):2815–20.

53. Kiprian D, Jarzabski A, Kawecki A. Evaluation of efficacy of Caphosol in prevention and alleviation of acute side effects in patients treated with radiotherapy for head and neck cancers. Contemp Oncol (Pozn) 2016;20(5):389–93.

54. Epstein JB, Epstein JD, Epstein MS, et al. Doxepin rinse for management of mucositis pain in patients with cancer: one week follow-up of topical therapy. Spec Care Dentist 2008;28(2):73–7.

55. Epstein JB, Saunders DP. Managing oral mucositis cancer therapy. 2015. Available at: http://www.oralhealthgroup.com/features/managing-oral-mucositis-cancer-therapy/. Accessed January 2, 2016.

56. Saunders DP, Epstein JB, Elad S, et al. Systematic review of antimicrobials, mucosal coating agents, anesthetics and analgesics for the management of oral mucositis in cancer patients. Support Care Cancer 2013;21:3191–207.

57. Bensadoun RJ, Riesenbeck D, Lockhart PB, et al. A systematic review of trismus induced by cancer therapies in head and neck cancer patients. Support Care Cancer 2010;18(8):1033–8.

58. Deng J, Ridner SH, Dietrich MS, et al. Prevalence of secondary lymphedema in patients with head and neck cancer. J Pain Symptom Manage 2012; 43(2):244–52.

59. Dijkstra PU, Kalk WW, Roodenburg JL. Trismus in head and neck oncology: a systematic review. Oral Oncol 2004;40(9):879–89.

60. Zecha JA, Raber-Durlacher JE, Nair RG, et al. Low-level laser therapy/photobiomodulation in the management of side effects of chemoradiation therapy in head and neck cancer: part 2: proposed applications and treatment protocols. Support Care Cancer 2016;24(6):2793–805.

61. Nederfors T. Xerostomia and hyposalivation. Adv Dent Res 2000;14:48–56.

62. Nutting CM, Morden JP, Harrington KJ, et al. Parotid-sparing intensity modulated versus conventional radiotherapy in head and neck cancer (PARSPORT): a phase 3 multicentre consensus controlled trial. Lancet Oncol 2011;12(2):127–36.

63. Dropcho EJ. Neurotoxicity of radiation therapy. Neurol Clin 2010;28(1):217–34.

64. Arduino PG, Porter SR. Oral and perioral herpes simplex virus type 1 (HSV-1) infection: review of its management. Oral Dis 2006;12(3):254–70.

65. Reusser P. Management of viral infections in immunocompromised cancer patients. Swiss Med Wkly 2002;132(27–28):374–8.

66. Lalla RV, Latortue MC, Hong CH, et al. A systematic review of oral fungal infections in patients receiving cancer therapy. Support Care Cancer 2010;18(8): 985–92.

67. Gøtzche PC, Johansen HK. Nystatin prophylaxis and treatment in severely immunocompromised patients. Cochrane Database Syst Rev 2002;(2): CD002033.

68. Worthington HV, Clarkson JE, Khalid T, et al. Interventions for treating oral candidiasis for patients with cancer receiving treatment. Cochrane Database Syst Rev 2010;(7):CD001972.

69. Lieshout HF, Bots CP. The effect of radiotherapy on dental hard tissue: a systematic review. Clin Oral Investig 2014;18(1):17–24.

70. Pyykonen H, Malmstrom M, Oikarinen VJ, et al. Late effects of radiation treatment of tongue and floor-of-mouth cancer on the dentition, saliva secretion, mucous membranes and the lower jaw. Int J Oral Maxillofac Surg 1986;15(4):401–9.

71. De Moor RJ, Stassen IG, van 't Veldt Y, et al. Two-year clinical performance of glass ionomer and resin composite restorations in xerostomic head-and-neck-irradiated cancer patients. Clin Oral Investig 2011;15(1):31–8.

72. Hey J, Seidel J, Schweyen R, et al. The influence of parotid gland sparing on radiation damages of dental hard tissues. Clin Oral Investig 2013;17(6): 1619–25.

73. Hey J, Setz J, Gerlach R, et al. Parotid gland-recovery after radiotherapy in the head and neck region: 36 months follow-up of a prospective clinical study. Radiat Oncol 2011;6:125.

74. Cohen EE, LaMonte SJ, Erb NL, et al. American Cancer Society head and neck cancer survivorship care guideline. CA Cancer J Clin 2016; 66(3):203–39.

75. Gomez DR, Estilo CL, Wolden SL, et al. Correlation of osteoradionecrosis and dental events with dosimetric parameters in intensity-modulated radiation therapy for head-and-neck cancer. Int J Radiat Oncol Biol Phys 2011;81(4):e207–13.

76. Dholam KP, Somani PP, Prabhu SD, et al. Effectiveness of fluoride varnish application as cariostatic and desensitizing agent in irradiated head and neck cancer patients. Int J Dent 2013;2013: 824982.

77. Thariat J, Ramus L, Darcourt V, et al. Compliance with fluoride custom trays in irradiated head and neck cancer patients. Support Care Cancer 2012; 20(8):1811–4.

78. Epstein JB, van der Meij E, Emerton S, et al. Compliance with fluoride gel use in irradiated patients. Spec Care Dentist 1995;15:218–22.

79. Epstein JB, McBride BC, Stevenson-Moore P, et al. The efficacy of chlorhexidine gel in reduction of Streptococcus mutans and Lactobacillus species in patients treated with radiation therapy. Oral Surg Oral Med Oral Pathol 1991;71:172–8.

80. Meca LB, Souza FR, Tanimoto HM, et al. Influence of preventive dental treatment on mutans streptococci counts in patients undergoing head and neck radiotherapy. J Appl Oral Sci 2009; 17(Suppl):5–12.

81. Pattni R, Walsh LJ, Marshall RI, et al. Changes in the periodontal status of patients undergoing bone marrow transplantation. J Periodontol 2000; 71(3):394–402.

82. Al-Nawas B, Grotz KA. Prospective study of the long term change of the oral flora after radiation therapy. Support Care Cancer 2006;14(3):291–6.

83. Nabil S, Samman N. Incidence and prevention of osteoradionecrosis after dental extraction in irradiated patients: a systematic review. Int J Oral Maxillofac Surg 2011;40(3):229–43.

84. Dhanda J, Pasquier D, Newman L, et al. Current concepts in osteoradionecrosis after head and neck radiotherapy. Clin Oncol (R Coll Radiol) 2016;28(7):459–66.

85. Chrcanovic BR, Reher P, Sousa AA, et al. Osteoradionecrosis of the jaws: a current overview. Part 1: physiopathology and risk and predisposing factors. Oral Maxillofac Surg 2010;14(1):3–16.

86. Reuther T, Schuster T, Mende U, et al. Osteoradionecrosis of the jaws as a side effect of radiotherapy of head and neck tumour patients: a report of a thirty year retrospective review. Int J Oral Maxillofac Surg 2003;32(3):289–95.

87. Sultan A, Hanna GJ, Margalit DN, et al. The use of hyperbaric oxygen for the prevention and management of osteoradionecrosis of the jaw: a Dana-Farber/Brigham and Women's Cancer Center multidisciplinary guideline. Oncologist 2017;22(3):343–50.

88. Delanian S, Depondt J, Lefaix JL. Major healing of refractory mandible osteoradionecrosis after treatment combining pentoxifylline and tocopherol: a phase II trial. Head Neck 2005;27(2):114–23.

89. Rivero JA, Shamji O, Kolokythas A. Osteoradionecrosis: a review of pathophysiology, prevention and pharmacologic management using pentoxifylline, a-tocopherol, and clodronate. Oral Surg Oral Med Oral Pathol Oral Radiol 2017;124:464–71.

90. Epstein JB, Hong PY, Ho AS, et al. Management of mucosal necrosis of the oropharynx in previously treated head and neck cancer patients. Support Care Cancer 2017;25:1031–4.

91. Hovan AJ, Williams PM, Stevenson-Moore P, et al. A systematic review of dysgeusia induced by cancer therapies. Support Care Cancer 2010; 18(8):1081–7.

92. Enriquez K, Lehrer E, Mullol J. The optimal evaluation and management of patients with a gradual onset of olfactory loss. Curr Opin Otolaryngol Head Neck Surg 2014;22(1):34–41.

93. Wrobel BB, Leopold DA. Olfactory and sensory attributes of the nose. Otolaryngol Clin North Am 2005;38(6):1163–70.

94. Holscher T, Seibt A, Appold S, et al. Effects of radiotherapy on olfactory function. Radiother Oncol 2005;77(2):157–63.

95. Sagar SM, Thomas RJ, Loverock LT, et al. Olfactory sensations produced by high-energy photon irradiation of the olfactory receptor mucosa in humans. Int J Radiat Oncol Biol Phys 1991;20(4): 771–6.

96. Buntzel J, Schuth J, Kuttner K, et al. Radiochemotherapy with amifostine cytoprotection for head and neck cancer. Support Care Cancer 1998; 6(2):155–60.

97. Komaki R, Lee JS, Milas L, et al. Effects of amifostine on acute toxicity from concurrent chemotherapy and radiotherapy for inoperable non-small-cell lung cancer: report of a randomized comparative trial. Int J Radiat Oncol Biol Phys 2004;58(5):1369–77.

98. Nagraj SK, Naresh S, Srinivas K, et al. Interventions for the management of taste disturbances. Cochrane Database Syst Rev 2014;(11):CD010470.

99. Ganzer H, Touger-Decker R, Byham-Gray L, et al. The eating experience after treatment for head and neck cancer: a review of the literature. Oral Oncol 2015,51(7):634–42.

100. Blanchard D, Bollet M, Dreyer C, et al. Management of somatic pain induced by head and neck cancer treatment: pain following radiation therapy and chemotherapy. Guidelines of the French Otorhinolaryngology Head and Neck Surgery Society (SFORL). Eur Ann Otorhinolaryngol Head Neck Dis 2014;131(4):253–6.

101. Mirabile A, Airoldi M, Ripamonti C, et al. Pain management in head and neck cancer patients undergoing chemo-radiotherapy: clinical practical recommendations. Crit Rev Oncol Hematol 2016;99:100–6.

102. Tan T, Barry P, Reken S, et al. Pharmacological management of neuropathic pain in non-specialist settings: summary of NICE guidance. BMJ 2010; 340:c1079.

103. Carvalho AL, Nishimoto IN, Califano JA, et al. Trends in incidence and prognosis for head and neck cancer in the United States: a site-specific analysis of the SEER database. Int J Cancer 2005;114(5):806–16.

104. Merkx MA, van Gulick JJ, Marres HA, et al. Effectiveness of routine follow-up of patients treated for

T1-2N0 oral squamous cell carcinomas of the floor of mouth and tongue. Head Neck 2006;28(1):1–7.

105. Deutschmann MW, Sykes KJ, Harbison J, et al. The impact of compliance in posttreatment surveillance in head and neck squamous cell carcinoma. JAMA Otolaryngol Head Neck Surg 2015;141(6):519–25.

106. Port JC, Farwell DG, Findlay M, et al. Optimal perioperative care in major head and neck surgery with free flap reconstruction: a consensus review and recommendations from the enhanced recovery surgery society. JAMA Otolaryngol Head Neck Surg 2017;143:292–303.

Head and Neck Cancer Research and Support Foundations

Joshua E. Lubek, MD, DDS

KEYWORDS

- Head and neck cancer research • Dysplasia • Immunotherapy • Xerostomia • Cancer organizations

KEY POINTS

- Ongoing genetic and epigenetic research involving DNA methylation, salivary biomarkers, wild-type p53 tumor suppressor gene proteins, and HPV oncogenes are being directed at identification and treatment of dysplastic and malignant squamous cell mucosal lesions.
- Research is being conducted to improve immunotherapy drug response rates by increasing the amount of inflammation within the tumor microenvironment.
- Ongoing research is focused on the application of the antidiabetic drug metformin for the prevention and management of oral squamous cell dysplastic lesions.
- The use of stem cells for the prevention and management of salivary dysfunction secondary radiotherapy is being investigated.
- Professional and nonprofit cancer support organizations are essential for furthering education and research within the area of head and neck cancer.

INTRODUCTION

The term head and neck cancer encompasses a large cohort of varied tumor pathologic conditions that can arise within the structures/subsites of the head and neck. Head and neck cancer ranks as the sixth most common type of cancer worldwide with head and neck squamous cell carcinoma (HNSCC) accounting for approximately 90% of all cases. It represents a significant global health concern because patients often present with advanced stage disease requiring extensive multimodality therapy (surgery, radiation, and chemotherapy). Patients often experience debilitating posttreatment side effects that affect quality of life as related to speech, swallowing, and cosmetic concerns. Many patients are unable to return to the workforce and are left on chronic disability.[1] Recurrence of disease is also of significant concern especially in those patients with advanced stage disease. The locoregional recurrence rates are approximately 40% with distant metastases occurring in 20% to 30% in this advanced stage cohort. This impact on patient recovery and function underscores the importance of both government and industry help to support research in the field of head and neck cancer. It also highlights the need for access to resources for patients and their families for their physical and emotional demands throughout their cancer care.

The vast number of research projects, published scientific abstracts/papers, and current clinical trials available within the discipline of head and neck cancer is obviously far too extensive to even attempt to summarize within this article of the *Oral and Maxillofacial Surgery Clinics of North America*. The purpose of this article is to provide

Disclosure: The author has nothing to disclose.
Oral–Head and Neck Surgery/Microvascular Surgery, Department of Oral and Maxillofacial Surgery, University of Maryland, 650 West Baltimore Street, Suite 1401, Baltimore, MD 21201, USA
E-mail address: jlubek@umaryland.edu

Oral Maxillofacial Surg Clin N Am 30 (2018) 459–469
https://doi.org/10.1016/j.coms.2018.06.007
1042-3699/18/© 2018 Elsevier Inc. All rights reserved.

a brief review of selected research topics in the specialty of HNSCC covering areas of cancer prevention, detection, surgical technologies, immunotherapy, genetics, and treatment sequelae. Various research foundations/resources available to those patients undergoing HNSCC and clinicians/researchers with an interest in HNSCC are also reviewed.

GENETIC AND EPIGENETIC RESEARCH

Numerous environmental events, such as the exposure to tobacco-associated carcinogens, ultraviolet light, and chronic viral infections, can result in both genetic and epigenetic changes leading to tumor development and disease progression. Genetic changes include events that lead to irreversible alterations in cellular DNA sequences, such as gene deletions, amplifications, and mutations, that damage tumor suppressor genes or activate oncogenes. Epigenetics refers to external modifications to DNA resulting in the inability for the cell to understand the genetic information. They are potentially reversible or transient modifications.[2–5]

DNA-methylation is one such epigenetic event that transfers a methyl group to the C-5 position of the cytosine ring of DNA by specific DNA-methyltransferases. The loss of heterozygosity of hypermethylated genes is often involved in tumor angiogenesis and the metastatic potential of HNSCC. Numerous hypermethylated genes identified within HNSCC involve cell-cycle control, programmed cell death, cell-cell interactions, and DNA repair mechanisms.

Tumor suppressor protein 53 (p53) responds to cell stress that arrests cell cycle and promotes DNA repair. Loss of p53 function results in human malignancy with more than 50% of observed HNSCC having p53 mutations identified within their cell DNA.

Methods of rapid, cost-effective identification of DNA-methylation patterns or p53 mutations are being studied to help identify potentially aggressive dysplastic lesions or in the use of intraoperative margin assessment. Brennan and colleagues[6] were the first group to identify p53 mutations using polymerase chain reaction (PCR) analysis at histologically negative surgical margins evaluated by pathologists using standard hematoxylin-eosin staining in a series of patients treated for oral squamous cell carcinoma. Interestingly, 38% of those with altered p53 mutations developed recurrence as compared with none without the mutation. This article was one of the first to explain why patients with so-called negative margins could develop local recurrence.

Limitations to the use of molecular markers of methylation for intraoperative margin assessment include the myriad of mutations that occur within a tumor creating difficulties in isolating those markers that are of highest risk for potential recurrence or transformation and the amount of time needed to analyze the data. Currently, no tests are available to be performed during the immediate operative procedure.[7]

Treatment of dysplasia and HNSCC through the use of gene therapy by introducing a wild-type p53 gene is currently under investigation. The wild-type p53 gene is an integral cancer suppressor gene that maintains genomic integrity by the production of a protein that arrests the cell cycle and stimulates DNA repair and cell apoptosis.

Introducing the p53 gene into the target cell is challenging. Viral vectors involve replacing a portion of the virus genome with a desired genetic sequence. The virus is injected into tumor cells and allowed to infect different cell types spreading the desired sequence. Of particular research interest is the use of modified adenoviruses. Adenoviruses are composed of DNA, unlike retroviruses, which are composed of RNA. Adenoviruses are not integrated into the host genome and do not cause any change to the host germ cell lineage.[8,9] One of the earliest research trials involving the use of gene therapy was described by Clayman and colleagues[10] in 1998, whereby the investigators injected an adenovirus vector p53 into 17 HNSCC patients with unresectable disease. Significant tumor response was reported in 47% of the cohort. A recent trial of advanced stage cervical cancer treated with recombinant human adenovirus-p53 and chemotherapy demonstrated a 95% efficacy with significant tumor shrinkage as compared with the chemotherapeutic arm.[11]

Routes of administration for recombinant adenovirus-p53 (rAD-p53) include intratumoral injection, perfusion, and intravenous injection. Good locoregional responses have been demonstrated in phase 2 trials for patients with HNSCC with combined radiotherapy and intratumoral rAD-p53. However, rAd-p53 alone has not been very successful in achieving complete responses. Intratumoral injection delivers the adenovirus to its target with good local effects and with less toxicity in comparison to the other routes of delivery. The spread of the rAD-p53 from the intratumoral injection site is limited, which limits its ability to affect more distant disease. Intra-arterial injection has been evaluated with good results; however, it does increase the risk of side effects, such as flulike symptoms and bone marrow suppression.[12,13] In a 2014 Chinese randomized placebo-controlled, double-blinded phase 3 trial consisting of 99 stage 3 and 4 patients with oral cancer, comparing intra-arterial infusion of combined rAD-p53 and chemotherapy versus chemotherapy alone demonstrated significantly increased survival rate in stage 3 patients but not in the stage 4 disease groups.[13] Other groups within the United States have been more skeptical because of poor patient accrual rates, regulatory hurdles, limited patient access to the research institutions, and mixed tumor response rates.[14] Despite these issues and mixed success, p53 gene therapy research continues, especially with a focus on delivery constructs: viral vectors, liposomes, cell-penetrating peptides, gold and magnetic nanoparticles, to increase the safety and efficacy of gene therapy.

IMMUNOTHERAPY

The first convincing proof as to the role of the immune system in cancer therapy was described by Muul and colleagues[15] in 1987, wherein the investigators noted the presence of a large number of tumor-infiltrating lymphocytes in skin melanoma and their cytolytic activity against malignant melanocytes when activated with interleukin-2 (IL-2). Immunotherapy research has been applied most notably to melanoma. Immunotherapy research has expanded the knowledge and understanding of the behavior of how malignant cells evade regulation by the immune system. Malignant cells, including HNSCC, can lose their specific antigens, thereby evading recognition by antigen-presenting cells. Alternatively, malignant cells may also express proteins that inhibit the immune system (downregulation) by stimulating immune checkpoints such as cytotoxic T-lymphocyte associated antigen-4 (CTLA-4), PD-1 (programmed death), and PD-L1 (programmed death ligand). Based on this scientific research, drugs, such as Ipilimumab (anti-CTLA-4), Nivolumab (anti-PD-1), and Pembrolizumab (anti-PD-1), have been developed.[16] Some of the earliest data in HNSCC were presented by Ferris and colleagues[17] in a randomized phase 3 trial (Checkmate-141) showing an improved overall 1-year survival in patients with advanced metastatic/platinum refractory HNSCC receiving Nivolumab versus cetuximab, docletaxol, or methotrexate. Newer drugs, such as Durvalumab (human immunoglobulin G1 antibody), that selectively inhibits PD-L1, is currently being investigated in several phase 1 HNSCC trials. There are challenges with the use of immunotherapy, including financial cost, autoimmune-related side effects, and tumor response rates. At least 50% to 60% of HNSCC express PD-L1; however, only a small fraction of those patients

(18% responders) will have a sustained meaningful response.[17] Current evidence suggests that there is increased upregulation of $CD8^+$ immunosuppression and PD-L1 in the inflamed tumor microenvironment (TME). Ongoing research to improve immunotherapy drug response rates by identifying tumors with a significantly inflamed TME is being conducted as evidenced by interferon-gamma (IFN-γ) production. Attempts to increase the inflammatory response within the TME with the use of attenuated viruses are also being investigated.[17–20] An example of this combined viral immunotherapy approach is the phase 1 multicenter, randomized trial using Talimogene laherparepvec in combination with pembrolizumab for recurrent or metastatic HNSCC (MASTERKEY232/KEYNOTE-137, NCT02626000).[21]

A working group sponsored by the National Cancer Institute has recommended groups of biomarkers for cancer immunotherapy to be collected, such as IFN-γ signatures, PD-1/PD-L1 expression, and serum-related cytokines and antibodies to be collected and analyzed for future microbiome studies. To date, none of these biomarkers have been validated in prospective trials.[22]

Immunotherapy drugs in HNSCC have potential as a therapeutic treatment arm. Currently, they are only approved in situations for advanced recurrent/metastatic disease in which patients have failed standard therapy because of the cost, limited clinical benefit, and potential immunologic side effects. There are limited clinical trials available investigating these drugs as primary therapy or for patients with high risk of recurrence. One such example involves a phase 2 trial of Pembrolizumab versus placebo in patients with head and neck cancer who are at high risk of recurrence following standard of care therapy (PATHWay study, NCT02841748). Another example includes the phase 1b trial investigating Ipilimumab in combination with intensity modulated radiotherapy (IMRT) and the epidermal growth factor receptor inhibitor Cetuximab (NCT03162731).[21]

DYSPLASIA
Detection and Surveillance

Oral cavity dysplasia describes the mucosal architectural changes with cytologic atypia found in the aerodigestive tract. Dysplasia occurs within a spectrum and is graded by the pathologist from mild dysplasia to severe dysplasia, involving the entire thickness of the squamous epithelium. Carcinoma in situ is designated once cellular malignant transformation has been identified but invasion has not violated the basement membrane into the underlying submucosal tissue. Treatment of these lesions, which often arise within white or white-red (leukoplakia/erythroleukoplakia) patches, vary widely between practitioners and can include observation, CO_2 laser ablation/excision, or formal excision with complete margin assessment. The ability to identify those patients whom require biopsy or treatment so as to prevent progression of disease or malignant transformation is an area of investigation. Currently, there are no specific markers identifying patients at highest risk of transformation.[23]

Noninvasive detection techniques are being tested to identify potentially malignant oral lesions and include vital stains, light-based detection, optical diagnostic technologies, and salivary biomarkers. The most common vital stains are Toluidine blue (binds dysplastic DNA) and Lugol's iodine (binds inversely to the glycogen uptake). They are useful but not diagnostic. These stains do not eliminate the need for biopsy, but may guide the clinician as to the best location for the highest yield biopsy or adjustment of a surgical margin during an ablative or excisional procedure.[23,24]

Light imaging techniques have low specificity because they cannot differentiate types of dysplasia.[24,25] In a study by Lane and colleagues,[26] despite a high rate of sensitivity and specificity reported by the authors, all lesions were identified by incandescent light. These noninvasive adjunctive techniques are still being investigated to optimize use and applicability. The best application may reside in the increased awareness of the health care practitioner performing the initial cancer screening or surveillance examination. Certainly, to rely exclusively on these adjunct noninvasive detection devices can lead to a false sense of security and does not replace thorough clinical evaluation.

Genetic alterations can be identified within bodily fluids that are associated with an affected organ. These alterations have led investigators to identify protein biomarkers within saliva, a readily accessible fluid for evaluation, in both premalignant and malignant disease states.[27–30] Newer amplification techniques via PCR evaluation and amplification assays have improved yields on appropriate identification and alleviated concerns about the use of saliva in contrast to serum. The limitation is in finding a cost-effective, rapid test with significant specificity. IL-6 and IL-8 have been studied because it is hypothesized that these inflammatory cytokines may play a role in the pathogenicity of oral squamous cell carcinoma (SCC). They can however be elevated in other inflammatory conditions, such as periodontal disease.[27,28]

Various microRNAs (miRNAs) are associated with overexpression, causing downregulation of tumor suppressor genes and underexpression resulting in oncogene upregulation. This aberrant overexpression can ultimately result in tumor occurrence or progression.[29,30] These miRNAs, which are readily accessible in saliva, are being investigated as a diagnostic screening method for the early detection of premalignant and malignant disease, assessing response to treatment and predicting prognosis or spread of disease. An example of this type of research is a recent study by Zahran and colleagues,[31] which evaluated 2 markers (miRNA-21 and miRNA-184) in patients with oral HNSCC and premalignant disease compared with normal controls. Zahran and colleagues found a 4-fold and 3-fold increase in miRNA levels respectively within their saliva. Sensitivity and specificity ranged from 65% to 75% and 65% to 80%, respectively. Concerns for the use of this tool involve the lack of well-matched clinical controls. Clinical trials are needed to identify normal expression of miRNAs and the quantity of expression in abnormal states.

Future applications of these tests could help in assessing risk of regional metastasis, thereby avoiding the need for elective neck dissection or sentinel node biopsy in patients with clinically N0 disease but deemed high risk for regional metastasis (ie, tumor depth greater than 3–4 mm in oral cavity SCC).[32]

Dysplasia and Metformin Treatment

Patients with field cancerization who develop multiple dysplasias with risk of progression of disease present a challenging problem for clinicians. Many cancer cells display the Warburg effect, a state of active glycolysis with lactate production under aerobic conditions.[33] The tumor cells consume glucose and release lactate. In vitro experiments have demonstrated that oral SCC can produce hypoxia-inducible factor 1α (HIF-1α) and increase ATP production through anaerobic glycolysis and induce oral SCC invasion. Various studies have suggested that the antidiabetic medication metformin may have antidysplastic effects or inhibitory effects on tumor proliferation. Experimental studies have demonstrated that metformin, a diabetic drug, can effectively inhibit HIF-1α activation in cells under hypoxia and thus inhibit cell proliferation and migration in an oral squamous cell model.[34–36] Indeed, metformin has also been associated with improved survival in clinical studies among HNSCC patients with diabetes.[37] In a recent small observational case series by Lerner and colleagues,[38] consisting of 3 nondiabetic patients with mucosal lesions and deemed high risk for recurrence, the patients showed a good response after being placed on metformin, not requiring further adjuvant therapy.

HUMAN PAPILLOMA VIRUS

Human papilloma virus (HPV) -induced carcinogenesis has become an extremely important topic of discussion as its role in the development of HNSCC becomes evident. Although HPV is clearly associated with oropharyngeal cancers, HPV is generally not a causal entity in HNSCC of the oral cavity SCC; indeed the reported incidence ranges from 4% to 6%.[39] Oropharyngeal SCC is now defined as having 2 very different types of disease behaviors. The classic pattern is linked to alcohol and tobacco, with patients presenting with advanced stage aggressive disease often requiring standard chemoradiotherapy with surgery reserved for salvage cases.[40] The HPV-induced pattern involves viral integration into the human cell leading to unregulated expression of HPV oncogenes that can inactivate tumor suppressor genes (ie, E6 inactivation of p53, E7 inactivates pRB). These HPV-related oropharyngeal cancers occur in non-smokers with a history of multiple sexual partners. Despite the fact that they present with more extensive nodal disease, they often fare better with improved long-term survival and decreased locoregional recurrence rates.[41] This difference in biologic behavior of HPV and non-HPV HNSCC is seen in the new American Joint Committee on Cancer (AJCC) staging system for oropharyngeal cancer, which changes the stage based on HPV status.

HNSCC research has focused greatly in the past decade on HPV-related HNSCC at all levels including: basic science/molecular, immune function, translational, and clinical research. These advances in research have significantly changed how we see and treat this disease. One of these areas of research includes immune modulating/vaccination. The prevalence of all HPV-associated malignancies is significant, 4.8% of all cancer worldwide.[42] Significant research has led to the development of 2 Food and Drug Administration (FDA) -approved vaccines against HPV. The quadrivalent HPV vaccine Gardasil covers the most common serotypes of HPV linked to cervical/oropharyngeal cancers (HPV type 16 and 18) and against serotypes HPV-6 and -11 linked to genital warts. A newer 9-valent vaccine (Gardasil 9) covers 5

additional HPV types that account for 15% of cervical cancers. The vaccinations are approved for girls and boys just before becoming sexually active and through the teenage years up to age 21. For those who have missed the vaccination and are in high-risk groups (HIV infection), it is approved up to age 26 years. Some of the earliest data to suggest the benefit were reported by Markowitz and colleagues,[43] in a study from 2003 to 2010, in which female young women aged 14 to 19 underwent cervicovaginal swabs. The incidence of HPV identified decreased by more than 50% in the group who had received the vaccination (HPV incidence 11.5% vs 5.1% in the vaccinated group). Public awareness campaigns and social media are needed to help improve the vaccination rates, because there are discrepancies within socioeconomic groups and gender, with regard to these vaccination rates. Interestingly, in a recent study by Choi and colleagues,[44] analyzing Centers for Disease Control and Prevention National Immunization Survey-Teen data, one of the most commonly cited parental reasons for not vaccinating their children was the absence of a recommendation by a health care provider (18%–25%). This finding clearly demonstrates that importance of the head and neck health care provider in providing education to the medical and dental community as to the potential long-term benefits of HPV vaccination.[45] Proof of the HPV vaccination campaign efficacy in the prevention of HPV-related oropharyngeal SCC will require years of data analysis because of the long latency period before the development of an HPV-related HNSCC.

Vaccine strategies are also being tested and applied to patients with HPV-related cancers in hopes of treatments and cure. Mutated HPV oncogenes E6 and E7 are being developed, allowing for an increased CD8[+] T-cell response in hopes to stimulate the immune system to destroy the tumor cells. Several studies have demonstrated significantly induced regression of E6/E7-expressing tumors in cervical cancer.[46]

With improved survival and disease-free recurrence related to HPV-associated oropharyngeal SCC continuing to increase, so too will the incidence of radiation-induced morbidities. Acute and late toxicities include mucositis, early and late dysphagia, atherosclerosis, hypothyroidism, and osteoradionecrosis (ORN). Surgery was generally limited as a salvage therapy, because it often required morbid access lip split mandibulotomy or pull-through approaches with flap reconstructive procedures. Recent technological advances in surgery have allowed more minimally invasive techniques such as transoral robotic surgery (TORS) to access and remove tumors of the oropharynx with the avoidance of those previously mentioned procedures.[47]

The recognition of the biologic behavior of HPV and the development of TORS has driven institutions and investigators to design trials to deescalate the intensity of oropharyngeal cancer treatment (both chemoradiation and surgery/radiation based), particularly in patients who are non-smokers with small burden disease (T1-2/N0-N1). Various national and international trials are underway, and patients should be encouraged to enroll in these trials because deescalation protocols have not yet been widely accepted as the standard of care.[48] Such trials include TORS with deintensified adjuvant radiotherapy, radiotherapy without chemotherapy, and deintensified radiotherapy doses (ie, ECOG 3311/NCT01898494).[21] Applications of such technology are being investigated for higher risk groups, such as in the HPV-negative population as well. A recent prospective study by Dabas and colleagues[49] evaluated patients who underwent TORS for T1-T2 HPV-negative oropharyngeal squamous cell carcinoma. Of the 49 patients with final pathologic stage I/II (AJCC 7th edition staging) disease, none received any adjuvant therapy, and disease-free survival (DFS) and overall survival (OS) were 89.6% and 93.8% at more than 2-years mean follow-up.

The initial TORS data are retrospective in nature and demonstrate similar DFS and OS rates. Criticism of a TORS-centric approach focuses on the need for adjuvant radiation in a significant portion of the TORS patients, presumably a contributing factor to the similar DFS and OS rates. A 2017 study by Monroe and colleagues[48] evaluating the Surveillance, Epidemiology, and End Results database of all patients who underwent TORS for pathologically confirmed T1-T2N1M0 patients were included in the evaluation. Of the 410 patients included, the 5-year OS and disease specific survival (DSS) were 77% and 86%, respectively. Radiation was administered in 74% of patients and was associated with a significantly improved OS. Limitations of the study include the lack of reporting on pathologic margin status, HPV status, and quality-of-life factors, such as dysphagia. Unfortunately, randomized controlled trials for the use of TORS and deintensification data are still pending. The likely benefit of TORS and other techniques of transoral resection for oropharyngeal HNSCC will be for small volume disease, where the avoidance or deescalation of adjuvant therapy reduces patient morbidity and decreases financial health care costs.[50,51]

COMPLICATIONS OF RADIOTHERAPY
Osteoradionecrosis

ORN is reported to occur in up to 15% of patients following radiotherapy treatment of HNSCC. Although radiotherapy techniques have greatly improved through intensity-modulated approaches (IMRT) and proton radiotherapy, ORN can be a significantly debilitating disease resulting in pain, foul odor, chronic infections, orocutaneous fistula, and pathologic fracture. Treatment can vary from conservative management and pain control for early stage disease or require surgical resection and microvascular flap reconstruction for advanced stage ORN.[52] Theories as to the pathophysiology behind this disease have included the Marx postulate (hypovascularity, hypoxia, hypocellularity) and the fibroatrophic theory (radiation-induced fibrosis by overactive fibroblast activity) as suggested by Delanian and Lefaix.[53,54] Various treatment regimens have focused on prevention and more conservative management, consisting of hyperbaric oxygen therapy, or medications, such as tocopherol and pentoxifylline, based on clinician philosophy as to pathophysiology. Regardless of treatment, once the patient develops significant necrosis, surgical resection with reconstruction becomes the primary method of management with overall good success.

Future directions of ORN research should focus on identification of patients at risk for ORN and prevention through counseling, prophylactic dental extraction, or possible medical therapy. The fibroatrophic theory of ORN suggests that excessive fibroblast activity modulated by transforming growth factor-beta 1 contributes to the stimulation and progression of the disease. Lyons and colleagues[55] identified a single nucleotide polymorphism in the promoter region of this gene that could predict which patients were at risk for ORN. The investigators isolated 3 alleles (CC, CT, TT) and identified that patients homozygous for the TT allele were at a 5.7 times odds risk for developing ORN after dentoalveolar treatment. A subsequent study on reconstructed patients identified higher risks of complications in patients with the TT allele, however, not statistically significant.[56] Regardless, these data points are worth future investigation to help counsel and possibly treat patients through future medications or gene therapy with the goal of prevention of this morbid complication of radiotherapy.

Mucositis and Xerostomia

Oral mucositis is a significant side effect of radiotherapy to the head and neck. It is an inflammatory response of the oropharyngeal mucosa with desquamation of the mucosa that can result in a painful debilitating condition that requires narcotics, alternative methods of nutrition, and prevention of infection. Although the risk is generally radiation dose dependent, there have been numerous salivary biomarkers studied to identify those patients at highest risk for the development of mucositis. It would be helpful to identify those patients, who may require more aggressive preventive measures during their radiation treatment. In a recent meta-analysis by Normando and colleagues,[57] an elevated epidermal growth factor, C-reactive protein, tumor necrosis-alpha, erythrocyte sedimentation rate, and abnormalities in the DNA repair genes $XRCC_1$, $XRCC_3$, and RAD 51 were associated with patients developing severe oral mucositis toxicities.

Salivary gland dysfunction as a result of external radiotherapy or radioactive iodine (^{131}I) can result in significant xerostomia with an incidence reported at approximately 70% to 80% of patients. The salivary gland damage is irreversible, with resulting problems including dental decay, tooth loss, infection, and dysphagia. Current treatments are aimed at symptomatic management or improvement in the function of remaining viable glandular tissue. Mesenchymal stem cells and human submandibular gland stem cells are currently being investigated because they have demonstrated the ability to migrate to glandular tissue and induce a repair process improving gland function and morphology. Currently, these experiments have only demonstrated success in the animal model.[58–61]

Other studies have focused on protecting or increasing salivary output. Xiang and colleagues[62] have studied phenylephrine to reduce radiosensitivity of the salivary glands through the nicotinamide phosphoribosyltransferase pathway. Other investigators are looking at pathways to protect damaged endothelial cells within the glands by targeting vascular endothelial proteins (vascular endothelial growth factor) and other endothelial reparative proteins.[63] Human aquaporin-1 is a plasma membrane protein that facilitates water movement across lipid membranes. Alevizos and colleagues[64–66] in 2017 published a small phase 1 trial using adenovirus-mediated transfer of the Aquaporin-1 gene in a series of 5 patients using the contralateral parotid gland as a control. All patients displayed increases in flow (>50%) with improved symptoms. A larger phase 1 study using an adenovirus vector encoding AQP-1 is recruiting for patients with established radiation-induced parotid dysfunction (NCT02446249).[21] These research endeavors are only a small example of the multiple efforts being made to improve the posttreatment quality of life.

SUPPORT FOUNDATIONS
www.clinicaltrials.gov

The ClinicalTrials.gov Web site is an informational Web site maintained by the National Library of Medicine at the National Institutes of Health. The purpose of the site is to provide information to patients, families, and clinicians regarding ongoing clinical human research based upon a protocol. Studies listed are conducted within the United States and 201 countries throughout the world. The FDA requires all studies involving a drug, biologic, or device be registered. Overall, the site is well organized, easily accessible, and easy to navigate. The user can enter desired key search words and all available studies will be listed. Accessing a specific study on the Web site will yield information regarding recruitment, purpose, inclusion/exclusion criteria, study details, and investigator and site contact information. In addition, there are links to relevant information, health Web sites, or other scientific papers (**Fig. 1**).

Professional and Patient-Centered Organizations

Head and neck cancer care cannot survive without various support foundations available through professional health care organizations or nonprofit charitable organizations. These organizations are integral in providing educational, emotional, and financial support to patients, families, and friends affected by head and neck cancer.

Not-for-profit organizations, such as The Oral Cancer Foundation (www.oralcancer.org) and the American Cancer Society (www.cancer.org), are available for the public to access freely and join as members. These organizations have similar missions of cancer care, including research, educational material, patient support, and patient care (disease prevention, detection, and treatment). Public awareness through social media, charitable events, and advertising campaigns help generate much needed financial dollars that are required for research grants and other patient support services. Such services include local oral cancer screenings and transportation assistance to and from medical appointments for those patients undergoing cancer care with limited financial and family support. Some of these organizations, such as the American Cancer Society, also sponsor peer-reviewed scientific journals for use by the health care community, for instance, *Cancer, CA: A Cancer Journal for Clinicians, Cancer Cytopathology* (**Fig. 2**).

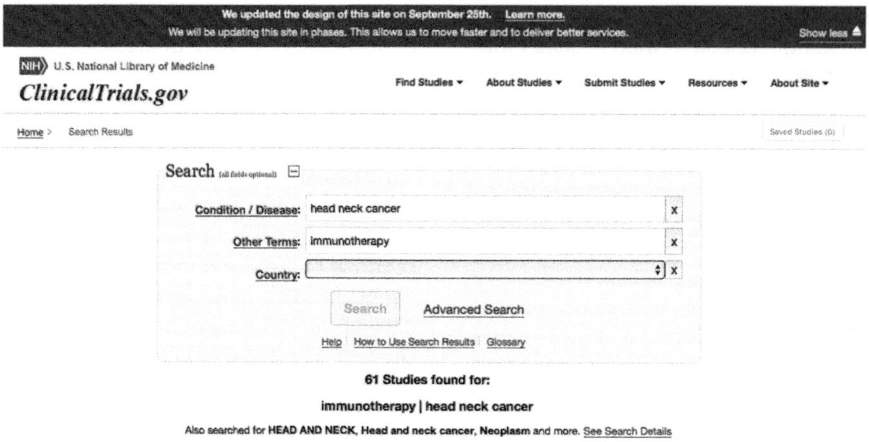

Fig. 1. Screenshot of the clinicaltrials.gov Web site homepage. (*Courtesy of* US National Library of Medicine, Bethesda, MD.)

This article cannot begin to list the numerous professional organizations and societies that are involved in public awareness campaigns, research, and education. These organizations and societies provide an incredibly valuable service by helping disseminate clinical information, often targeting both the layperson and the health care professional. Their mission ultimately improves the quality of head and neck cancer care. Examples of such organizations include the American Association of Oral Maxillofacial Surgery (www.aaoms.org), the American Dental Association (www.ADA.org), the American Head and Neck Society (www.AHNS.info), and the National Comprehensive Cancer Network (www.nccn.org).

Two professional organizations improve the quality of care delivered by helping standardize the staging and treatment guidelines for cancer. The National Comprehensive Cancer Network is a nonprofit alliance of 27 cancer centers in the United States (designated by the National Cancer Institute) devoted to patient education and improvement of quality patient care. The network publishes a peer-reviewed scientific titled the *Journal of the National Comprehensive Cancer Network*. Membership is free, and patients and clinicians are able to access the clinical guidelines. The treatment guidelines and recommendations are separated for the various head and neck cancer subsites and are based on current and outcome-based research. These guidelines are updated and based on consensus data reviewed by a multidisciplinary group of experts within each oncologic subsite.

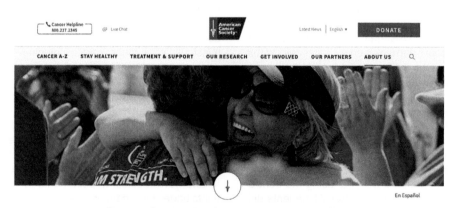

About the American Cancer Society

At the American Cancer Society, we're on a mission to free the world from cancer. Until we do, we'll be funding and conducting research, sharing expert information, supporting patients, and spreading the word about prevention. All so you can live longer — and better.

Fig. 2. Screenshot of the American Cancer Society Web site homepage (cancer.org). *Reprinted by* the permission of the American Cancer Society, Inc. www.cancer.org. All rights reserved.

The AJCC (www.cancerstaging.org) is an organization dedicated to cancer research, care, and education. Currently, there are 22 member organizations affiliated with the AJCC (ie, American College of Surgeons). All of these affiliate organizations continue to have significant involvement in the field of cancer, such as epidemiology, patient care, prevention, education, and research. One of the most significant contributions to cancer research by the AJCC was in developing a comprehensive cancer staging system for all cancers of the body (TNM) that helps to guide patient plan of care treatment based on epidemiologic and collected treatment data reviewed by expert panels and committees. The new AJCC 8th edition staging system for head and neck cancers is to be implemented for 2018.[67]

REFERENCES

1. Wissinger E, Griebsch I, Lungershausen J, et al. The economic burden of head and neck cancer: a systematic literature review. Pharmacoeconomics 2014;32:865–82.
2. Khan SS, Kamboj M, Verma R, et al. Epigenetics in oral cancer- neoteric biomarker. J Oral Med Oral Surg Oral Pathol Oral Radiol 2016;2:62–5.
3. Goldberg AD, Allis CD, Bernstein E. Epigenetics: a landscape takes shape. Cell 2007;128:635–8.
4. Holliday R. Epigenetics: a historical overview. Epigenetics 2006;1:76–80.
5. Hema KN, Smitha T, Sheethal HS, et al. Epigenetics in oral squamous cell carcinoma. J Oral Maxillofac Pathol 2017;21:252–9.
6. Brennan JA, Mao L, Hruban RH, et al. Molecular assessment of histopathological staging in squamous cell carcinoma of the head and neck. N Engl J Med 1995;332:429–35.
7. Clark DJ, Mao L. Understanding the surgical margin:a molecular assessment. Oral Maxillofac Surg Clin North Am 2017;29:245–58.
8. Ajith TA. Strategies used in the clinical trials of gene therapy for cancer. J Exp Ther Oncol 2017;11:33–9.
9. Nemunaitis J, Nemunaitis J. Head and neck cancer: response to p53-based therapeutics. Head Neck 2011;33:131–4.
10. Clayman GL, el-Naggar AK, Lippman SM, et al. Adenovirus-mediated p53 genetransfer in patients with advanced recurrent head and neck squamous cell carcinoma. J Clin Oncol 1998;16:2221–32.
11. Xiao J, Zhou J, Min F, et al. Efficacy of recombinant human adenovirus-p53 combined with chemotherapy for locally advanced cervical cancer: a clinical trial. Oncol Lett 2017;13:3676–80.
12. Zhang SW, Xiao SW, Liu CQ, et al. Treatment of head and neck squamous cell carcinoma by recombinant adenovirus-p53 combined with radiotherapy: a phase II clinical trial of 42 cases. Zhonghua Yi Xue Za Zhi 2003;83:2023–8.
13. Li Y, Li LJ, Wang LJ, et al. Selective intra-arterial infusion of rAD-p53 with chemotherapy for advanced oral cancer: a randomized clinical trial. BMC Med 2014;12:16.
14. Yoo GH, Moon J, LeBlanc M, et al. A phase II trail of surgery with perioperative INGN 201(Ad5CMV-p53) gene therapy followed by chemoradiotherapy for advanced resectable squamous cell carcinoma of the oral cavity, oropharynx, hypopharynx and larynx; report of the southwest oncology group. Arch Otolaryngol Head Neck Surg 2009;135:869–74.
15. Muul LM, Spiess PJ, Director EP, et al. Identification of specific cytolytic immune responses against autologous tumor in humans bearing malignant melanoma. J Immunol 1987;138:989–95.
16. Rotte A, Jin JY, Lemaire V. Mechanistic overview of immune checkpoints to support the rational design of their combinations in cancer immunotherapy. Ann Oncol 2017. https://doi.org/10.1093/annonc/mdx686.
17. Ferris RL, Blumenschein J Jr, Fayette J, et al. Nivolumab for recurrent squamous cell carcinoma of the head and neck. N Engl J Med 2016;375:1856–67.
18. Concha-Benavente F, Srivasrava RM, Trivedi S, et al. Identification of the cell-intrinsic and extrinsic pathways downstream of EGFR and IFNγ that induce PD-L1 expression in head and neck cancer. Cancer Res 2016;76:1031–43.
19. Ayers M, Lunceford J, Nebozhyn M, et al. IFN-gamma related mRNA profile predicts clinical response to PD-1 blockade. J Clin Invest 2017;127:2930–40.
20. Kumai T, Fan A, Harabuchi Y, et al. Cancer immunotherapy: moving forward with peptide T cell vaccines. Curr Opin Immunol 2017;47:57–63.
21. U.S. National Library of Medicine, Available at: www.ClinicalTrials.gov. Accessed October 1, 2017.
22. Bauman JE, Cohen E, Ferris RL, et al. Immunotherapy of head and neck cancer: emerging clinical trials from a national cancer institute head and neck cancer steering committee planning meeting. Cancer 2017;123:1259–71.
23. Kumar A, Cascarini L, McCaul JA, et al. How should we manage oral leukoplakia? Br J Oral Maxillofac Surg 2013;51:377–83.
24. Awan KH, Morgan PR, Warnakulasuriya S. Assessing the accuracy of autofluoresescence, chemiluminescence and toluidine blue as diagnostic tools for oral potentially malignant disorders- a clinicopathological evaluation. Clin Oral Investig 2015;19:2267–72.
25. Awan KH, Morgan PR, Warnakulasuriya S. Evaluation of an autofluorescence based imaging system (VELscope) in the detection of oral potentially

malignant disorders and benign keratoses. Oral Oncol 2011;47:274–7.

26. Lane PM, Gilhuly T, Whitehead P, et al. Simple device for the direct visualization of oral-cavity tissue fluorescence. J Biomed Opt 2006;11(2): 024006.

27. Chen Z, Malhotra PS, Thomas GR, et al. expression of proinflammatory and proangiogenic cytokines in patients with head and neck cancer. Clin Cancer Res 1999;5:1369–79.

28. St John MA, Li Y, Zhou X, et al. Interleukin 6 and interleukin 8 as potential biomarkers for oral cavity and oropharyngeal squamous cell carcinoma. Arch Otolaryngol Head Neck Surg 2004;130:929–35.

29. Momen-Heravi F, Trachtenberg AJ, Kuo WP, et al. Genomwide study of salivary microRNAs for detection of oral cancer. J Dent Res 2014;93:86S–93S.

30. Chen CZ. MicroRNAs as oncogenes and tumor suppressors. N Engl J Med 2005;353:1768–71.

31. Zahran F, Ghalwash D, Shaker O, et al. Salivary microRNAs in oral cancer. Oral Dis 2015;21:739–47.

32. Abu-Ghanem S, Yehuda M, Carmel NN, et al. Elective neck dissection vs observation in early stage squamous cell carcinoma of the oral tongue with no clinically apparent lymph node metatstasis in the neck a systematic review and meta analysis. JAMA Otolaryngol Head Neck Surg 2016;142: 857–65.

33. Warburg O. On the origin of cancer cells. Science 1956;123:309–14.

34. Fraga CA, Sousa AA, Correa GT, et al. High hypoxia-inducible factor-1 alpha expression genotype associated with eastern cooperative oncology group performance in head and neck squamous cell carcinoma. Head Neck Oncol 2012;4:77.

35. Fraga CA, de Oliveria MV, de Oliveria ES, et al. A high HIF-1 alpha expression genotype is associated with poor prognosis of upper aerodigestive tract carcinoma patients. Oral Oncol 2012;48: 130–5.

36. Guimaraes TA, Farias LC, Santos ES, et al. Metformin increases PDH and suppresses HIF-1 alpha under hypoxic conditions and induces cell death in oral squamous cell carcinoma. Oncotarget 2016;7: 55057–68.

37. Rego DF, Pavan LM, Elias ST, et al. Effects of metformin on head and neck cancer: a systematic review. Oral Oncol 2015. https://doi.org/10.1016/j.oraloncology.2015.01.007.

38. Lerner MZ, Mor N, Paek H, et al. Metformin prevents the progression of dysplastic mucosa of the head and neck to carcinoma in nondiabetic patients. Ann Otol Rhinol Laryngol 2017;126:340–3.

39. Herrero R, Castellsague X, Pawlita M, et al. Human papillomavirus and oral cancer: the international agency for research on cancer multicenter study. J Natl Cancer Inst 2003;95:1772–83.

40. Chaturvedi AK, Engels EA, Pfeiffer RM, et al. Human papillomavirus and rising oropharyngeal cancer incidence in the United States. J Clin Oncol 2011; 29:4294–301.

41. Fakhry C, Westra WH, Li S, et al. Improved survival of patients with human papillomavirus positive head and neck squamous cell carcinoma in a prospective clinical trial. J Natl Cancer Inst 2008;100: 261–9.

42. de Martel C, Ferlay J, Franceschi S, et al. Global burden of cancers attributable to infections in 2008: a review and synthetic analysis. Lancet Oncol 2012;13:607–15.

43. Markowitz LE, Dunne EF, Saraiya M, et al. Human papillomavirus vaccination: recommendations of the advisory committee on immunization practices (ACIP). MMWR Recomm Rep 2014;63:1–30.

44. Choi Y, Eworuke E, Segal R. What explains the different rates of human papillomavirus vaccination among adolescent males and females in the United States? Papillomavirus Res 2016;2:46–51.

45. Kasting ML, Scherr CL, Ali KN, et al. Human papillomavirus vaccination training experience among family medicine residents and faculty. Fam Med 2017; 49:714–22.

46. Li J, Chen S, Ge J, et al. A novel therapeutic vaccine composed of a rearranged human papillomavirus type 16 E6/E7 fusion protein and Fms-like tyrosine kinase-3 ligand induces CD8+ T cell responses and antitumor effect. Vaccine 2017;35:6459–67.

47. Adelstein DJ, Ridge JA, Brizel DM, et al. Transoral resection of the pharyngeal cancer: summary of a national cancer institute head and neck cancer steering committee clinical trials planning meeting, November 6-7, 2011, Arlington Virginia. Head Neck 2012;34:1681–703.

48. Monroe MM, Buchmann LO, Hunt JP, et al. The benefit of adjuvant radiation in surgically-treated T1-2 N1 oropharyngeal squamous cell carcinoma. Laryngoscope Investig Otolaryngol 2017;2:57–62.

49. Dabas S, Gupta K, Ranjan R, et al. Oncological outcome following de-intensification of treatment for stage I and II HPV negative oropharyngeal cancers with transoral robotic surgery (TORS); a prospective trial. Oral Oncol 2017;69:80–3.

50. Weistein GS, O'malley BW, Magnuson JS, et al. Transoral robotic surgery: a multicenter study to assess feasibility, safety and surgical margins. Laryngoscope 2012;122:1701–7.

51. Richmon JD, Quon H, Gourin CG. The effect of transoral robotic surgery on short term outcomes and cost of care after oropharyngeal cancer surgery. Laryngoscope 2014;124:165–71.

52. Lubek JE, Hancock MK, Strome SE. What is the value of hyperbaric oxygen therapy in the management of osteoradionecrosis of the head and neck? Laryngoscope 2013;123:555–6.

53. Marx RE. Osteoradionecrosis; a new concept of its pathophysiology. J Oral Maxillofac Surg 1983;41: 283–8.

54. Delanian S, Lefaix JL. The radiation-induced fibroatrophic process: therapeutic perspective via the antioxidant pathway. Radiother Oncol 2004;73: 119–31.

55. Lyons AJ, West CM, Risk J, et al. Osteoradionecrosis in head and neck cancer has a distinct genotype-dependent cause. Int J Radiat Oncol Biol Phys 2012;82:1479–84.

56. Lyons AJ, Nixon I, Papadopoulou D, et al. Can we predict which patients are likely to develop severe complications following reconstruction for osteoradionecrosis? Br J Oral Maxillofac Surg 2013;51: 707–13.

57. Normando AGC, Rocha CL, de Toledo IP, et al. Biomarkers in the assessment of oral mucositis in head and neck cancer patients: a systematic review and meta-analysis. Support Care Cancer 2017;25: 2969–88.

58. Jensen SB, Pedersen AM, Vissinik A, et al. A systematic review of salivary gland hypofunction and xerostomia induced by cancer therapies: prevalence, severity and impact on quality of life. Support Care Cancer 2010;18:1039–60.

59. Nevens D, Nuyts S. The role of stem cells in the prevention and treatment of radiation induced xerostomia in patients with head and neck cancer. Cancer Med 2016;5:1147–53.

60. Lombaert IM, Wiernga PK, Kok T, et al. Mobilization of bone marrow stem cells by granulocyte colony-stimulating factor ameliorates radiation induced damage to salivary glands. Clin Cancer Res 2006; 12:1804–12.

61. Lim JY, Ra JC, Shin IS, et al. Systemic transplantation of human adipose tissue derived mesenchymal stem cells for the regeneration of irradiation induced salivary gland damage. PLoS One 2013;8(8): e71167.

62. Xiang B, Han L, Wang X, et al. Nicotinamide phosphoribosyltransferase upregulation by phenylephrine reduces radiation injury in submandibular gland. Int J Radiat Oncol Biol Phys 2016;96:538–46.

63. Mizrachi A, Cotrim AP, Katabi N, et al. Radiation induced microvascular injury as a mechanism of salivary gland hypofunction and potential target for radioreceptors. Radiat Res 2016;186:189–95.

64. Alevizos I, Zheng C, Cotrim AP. Late responses to adenoviral-mediated transfer of the aquaporin-1 gene for radiation induced salivary hypofunction. Gene Ther 2017;24:176–86.

65. Verma V, Simone CB 2nd, Mishra MV. Quality of life and patient reported outcomes following proton radiation therapy: a systematic review. J Natl Cancer Inst 2018;110(4). https://doi.org/10.1093/jnci/djx208.

66. Phan J, Sio TT, Nguyen TP, et al. Reirradiation of head and neck cancers with proton therapy: outcomes and analyses. Int J Radiat Oncol Biol Phys 2016;1:30–41.

67. Amin MB, Edge S, Greene F, et al, editors. AJCC cancer staging manual. 8th edition. Springer; 2017.

Physical Rehabilitation and Occupational Therapy

Lauren C. Capozzi, MD, PhD[a],*, Naomi D. Dolgoy, OT[b], Margaret L. McNeely, PT, PhD[c]

KEYWORDS

- Physical activity • Physical therapy • Occupational therapy • Exercise • Rehabilitation
- Head and neck cancer

KEY POINTS

- Head and neck cancer can lead to dysfunction and disfigurement, affecting the physical function and quality of life of patients.
- The American Cancer Society's Head and Neck Survivorship Care Guidelines recommend a full rehabilitation assessment of all patients after their treatments to manage many of the complications that may impact long-term recovery and function.
- Evidence supports the role of physical activity and exercise as an important rehabilitation tool that can improve strength, endurance, physical function, and quality of life, and decrease symptom burden after surgery and other treatments.
- Physical therapy techniques help to optimize jaw, neck, and shoulder function.
- Occupational therapy techniques help to enhance quality of life through modified activities and improved return to work outcomes.

INTRODUCTION

Patients with head and neck cancer (HNC) can become debilitated directly by disease and secondarily by treatment, which affect structures and function in the head and neck region, as well as other body sites and systems. The results often lead to local and regional disfigurement and dysfunction. Inherently, this disease and its associated treatment also impact psychosocial as well as physical aspects of function in patients.[1–3] With advancements in early detection, tumor characterization, and management, emerging evidence supports the role of rehabilitation to improve the physical and psychosocial function of patients once diagnosed.[4] The changing epidemiology of HNC posed by the increasing incidence of cancers associated with the human papillomavirus has resulted in a younger average age at diagnosis and an improved rate of response to treatment.[5] With more patients surviving after treatment of HNC, strategies to improve patient function are more important than ever.

In 2016, the American Cancer Society published the Head and Neck Cancer Survivorship Care Guidelines and outlined recommendations for the rehabilitation of patients with HNC after treatments.[6] The guidelines specifically recommend that primary care providers, including the primary oncologist, assess patients for spinal accessory nerve (SAN) palsy, cervical dystonia and muscle spasms, neuropathies, shoulder dysfunction, trismus, postoperative lymphedema, weight management, fatigue, sleep disturbance, self-image concerns, depression, and anxiety. As indicated,

Disclosure: The authors have nothing to disclose.
[a] Division of Physical Medicine and Rehabilitation & Faculty of Medicine, Cumming School of Medicine, Foothills Medical Centre, 1403-29 Street NW, Calgary, Alberta T2N 2T9, Canada; [b] Faculty of Rehabilitation Medicine, University of Alberta, 2-50 Corbett Hall, Edmonton, Alberta T6G 2G4, Canada; [c] Faculty of Rehabilitation Medicine, University of Alberta, Cross Cancer Institute, 2-50 Corbett Hall, Edmonton, Alberta T6G 2G4, Canada
* Corresponding author.
E-mail address: lcapozzi@ucalgary.ca

Oral Maxillofacial Surg Clin N Am 30 (2018) 471–486
https://doi.org/10.1016/j.coms.2018.06.008
1042-3699/18/© 2018 Elsevier Inc. All rights reserved.

patients should be referred to appropriate physical therapists, occupational therapists, or exercise specialists for rehabilitation programs. The guidelines also recommend that patients with HNC should be counseled on regular participation in physical activity in accordance with public health guidelines to achieve 150 minutes of moderate or 75 minutes of vigorous aerobic activity per week, plus strength training at least 2 days per week (**Box 1**).[6]

Despite increasing evidence and clear recommendations that support the role of rehabilitation in patients with cancer, the clinical support and resources remain lacking for patients to undergo efforts before and after treatment. The inability to access care for rehabilitation results in functional decline that brings to bear longer recovery time, impaired quality of life, and increased health care costs. Not only is rehabilitation critical to the recovery of patients after cancer treatment, it is also cost effective.[9] Translating evidence-based guidelines for rehabilitation into clinical practice offers an effective and valuable opportunity to improve outcomes in patients with HNC.

This chapter presents the unique physical challenges faced by survivors of HNC and specific interventions of rehabilitation that are supported by a growing body of evidence. Exercise therapy strategies to boost physical and psychosocial functioning, as well as specific physical therapy (PT) and occupational therapy (OT) for patients in this unique population are also discussed.

Box 1
Physical activity guidelines for cancer survivors

Based on the American Counsel of Sports Medicine Roundtable meeting on

Exercise for Cancer Survivors[7] and American Cancer

Society's Guidelines for Cancer Survivors[8]

- 150 minutes of moderate intensity aerobic exercise or 75 minutes of vigorous aerobic exercise per week
- 2 to 3 days of strength training per week
- Flexibility training on most days of the week
- Overall, avoid inactivity and return to daily activities as soon as possible

Data from Rock CL, Doyle C, Demark-Wahnefried W, et al. Nutrition and physical activity guidelines for cancer survivors. CA Cancer J Clin 2012;62(4):243–74; and Schmitz KH, Courneya KS, Matthews C, et al. American College of Sports Medicine roundtable on exercise guidelines for cancer survivors. Med Sci Sports Exerc 2010;42(7):1409–26.

HEAD AND NECK CANCER: SPECIFIC CHALLENGES AND THE ROLE FOR REHABILITATION

HNC and related treatments can affect the bones, joints, muscles, glands, lymphatics, and neurovascular tissue in patients, impairing vital functions of respiration, auditory, olfactory, and gustatory sensation, mastication, and communication. Muscle or nerve damage can also effect the musculoskeletal function of the cervical and thoracic spine and shoulders, causing persistent pain and difficulties with activities of daily living (ADLs).

Although surgery specifically aims to remove tumor and ameliorate some of the physical and functional implications related to the tumor extent, complications commonly affect soft tissues and organs, such as SAN palsy, cervical dystonia, cervical neuropathies, and shoulder dysfunction. Additional effects may include impaired oral function, airway patency, mastication, and speech. The removal of lymphatic tissue may result in lymphedema of the face and neck region. Many patients report ongoing fatigue, which may be related to deconditioning, loss of lean muscle mass, and sleep disturbance. Finally, the physical and functional changes that occur after surgery can profoundly impact body image and mood. Fortunately, rehabilitation can compensate for the detrimental side effects of surgery, as well as the cancer-fighting therapies of radiation and chemotherapy, to help patients recover after treatment of cancer. These challenges and the associated pathophysiology—the physical, psychological, and functional impacts—and the rehabilitation recommendations are summarized in **Table 1**.

PHYSICAL ACTIVITY AND EXERCISE FOR THE PATIENT WITH HEAD AND NECK CANCER

Importantly, physical activity, or overall body movement, is differentiated from exercise, a subset of physical activity that is intended for rehabilitation and health benefit.[20] In this section, we discuss the role for overall physical activity and the specific role for exercise as a therapy in prehabilitation and rehabilitation.

Evidence supporting the benefit of overall activity for survivors of HNC has grown substantially over the last 15 to 20 years.[7] Clearly, physical activity plays an important part in preparing patients to withstand difficult treatments and to recover after treatment.[7] The physical and psychosocial benefits of physical activity are summarized in **Table 2**. Moreover, improved outcomes in survival with reduced rates of recurrence, cancer-specific

Table 1
Specific challenges in head and neck cancer and the role for rehabilitation

Challenges	Pathophysiology	Physical Impact – Disfigurement and Dysfunction	Psychosocial Impact	Impact on Overall Function	Rehabilitation Recommendations
Spinal accessory nerve palsy and associated shoulder dysfunction	Damage to cranial nerve XI, responsible for innervation of trapezius and sternocleidomastoid muscles[10]	• Shoulder pain and limited ROM (ie, decreased abduction) • Neck pain and limited ROM (ie, lateral flexion and rotation) • Scapular winging • Atrophy and associated weakness of the trapezius	• Difficulty with work and role function[6] • Physical impairment is associated with increased anxiety and depression	• Decreased ROM, resulting in limited ability to complete independent activities of daily living, such as reaching over-head to dress or shower[11] • Excessive use, resistance, or weight bearing can lead to adhesive capsulitis	• Referral to a rehabilitation specialist for ROM and progressive strengthening[6] • Rehabilitative interventions for functional mobility, clothing adaptation, instrumental/activities of daily living modifications[11] • Education regarding load distribution, carrying techniques to avoid nerve compression
Cervical dystonia - torticollis	Repetitive spasms of the cervical muscles owing to neuromuscular dysfunction after surgery or radiation[12]	• Ongoing pain, cramping, involuntary muscle movements, limited neck ROM • Compensatory posturing leading to pain and functional impairment of the other upper extremity and back	• Pain can be disabling, leading to anxiety and depression	• Barriers to managing basic daily activities • Fatigue can result in deconditioning, and reduction of activity participation	• Nerve stabilizing agents, including pregabalin, gabapentin, duloxetine, or botulinum toxin type A injections • Functional interventions for instrumental/activities of daily living[13]

(continued on next page)

Table 1
(continued)

Challenges	Pathophysiology	Physical Impact – Disfigurement and Dysfunction	Psychosocial Impact	Impact on Overall Function	Rehabilitation Recommendations
Cervical neuropathies	Paresthesia from nerve damage after surgical and radiological interventions[6]	• Can impact sensory and motor function, leading to changes in dexterity, grasp, and sensation[11] • May lead to paresthesia	• Pain can be exhausting and disabling, leading to anxiety, depression and decreased QOL[14]	• Difficulties with instrumental/activities of daily living • Difficulties with complex upper extremity tasks • Increased risk for upper extremity injuries (burns and frostbite), and wounds	• Nerve stabilizing agents, including pregabalin, gabapentin, duloxetine or botulinum toxin type A injections • Neuromuscular reeducation and sensory retraining
Trismus	Characterized by reduced jaw ROM (<35 mm) owing to damage to the soft tissues from surgery or radiation therapy[15]	• Difficulties with mouth opening, eating limitations, muscular tension, dry mouth, and pain with swallowing	• Negative impact on health-related QOL, increased rates of depression and pain	• Difficulties with chewing, swallowing, and managing oral hygiene • Challenges with oral communication and facial expressions	• Refer to dental professionals for prevention and treatment • Treat with nerve stabilizing agents as necessary • Maxillofacial exercises for managing limited jaw opening • Modified/adapted devices, equipment
Lymphedema	Edema, or swelling, caused by the inability of the lymphatic system to absorb interstitial fluid[6]	• Swelling to the face and/or neck • Can result in changes to tissue, and increase risks of wounds and cellulitis[16] • Can impact swallowing and jaw mobility	• Chronic nature of lymphedema and related physical impairments can lead to feelings of loss and psychoemotional challenges[16]	• Can impact activities of daily living, including oral hygiene and self-feeding • Environment, weather, and position can impact edema	• Complete decongestive therapy, which includes skin care, manual lymph drainage, and compression techniques[6]

Fatigue (cancer related)	• Persistent, highly distressing consequence of cancer and its treatments that negatively impacts all domains of life • Complex pathology, including neurologic and physical causes[17]	• Decrease endurance and ability to carry out tasks	• Correlations with depression and anxiety	• Fluctuating and unpredictable presentation • Difficulty planning daily routines, and participating in tasks	• Evidence supports exercise as a key fatigue management strategy • Functional rehabilitation supporting goal setting, energy maximization, activity prioritization, and grading/adapting activities[11]
Mood disturbance: depression, anxiety and body image disturbance	• Decreased QOL and daily function correlates with increased rates of stress, anxiety, worry, thoughts of depression, loss and grief[18]	• Can impact PA participation, energy levels, and overall attitude toward wellness	• Psychological well-being decreases with increased anxiety, depression and body image disturbance	• Low mood states and high stress or worry states can be detrimental to activity engagement • Withdrawal and social isolation often accompany mood issues	• PA improves mood by decreasing reported anxiety, depression, body image disturbance and feelings of control
Weight management/management of cancer cachexia and deconditioning	• Patients with HNC are at increased risk for cachexia and weight loss • Up to 70% of weight loss can be related to muscle wasting[9]	• Changes to body composition, specifically weight loss related to burden of disease, cachexia, and changes to appetite and physical ability to eat can impact overall physical function[19]	• Illness-related weight changes often correlate with reduced QOL	• Increased difficulty managing energy levels and keeping up with physical demands of work or activities of daily living[17] • Higher risk for falls, decreased functioning, increased disease burden[11]	• Progressive resistance training plays a key role in maintaining or regaining skeletal muscle after treatment • Eating at set times, and after listed meal guidelines as determined through dietetics referral

Abbreviations: PA, physical activity; QOL, quality of life; ROM, range of motion.

Table 2
Physical and psychosocial benefits of physical activity for patients with head and neck cancer[a]

	Physical	Psychosocial
Increase	Weight management Lean body mass Upper and lower body strength Lower body endurance Aerobic functioning Postural stability Physical and functional well-being Appetite Associated with improved survival	Overall quality of life Social well-being Cognition (Samuel et al,[25] 2013) Emotional well-being Vitality
Decrease	Tiredness and drowsiness Reliance on feeding tube at 1 year	Pain Depression Anxiety Distress

[a] Based on observational and randomized trials.

Data from Capozzi LC, Nishimura KC, McNeely ML, et al. The impact of physical activity on health related fitness and quality of life for head and neck cancer patients: a systematic review. Br J Sports Med 2016;50(6):325–38.

and non–cancer-specific mortality have been recently found in cancer survivors who increased their activity level after diagnosis.[21,22] Physical activity has also been found to improve fitness outcomes including strength, endurance, and aerobic capacity, and to improve physical functioning outcomes and psychosocial factors by decreasing depression, anxiety, and sleep difficulties.[21,23] Individuals who participate in an activity program after diagnosis are more likely to return to work and in less time.[24] Based on the work of the American Counsel of Sports Medicine, 150 minutes of moderate intensity activity, plus 2 to 3 days of strength training per week is recommended for everyone living with cancer (see **Box 1**).[21] The same recommendation has been supported by the American Cancer Society and the World Health Association.[8]

The investigation of physical activity and structured exercise programming for patients with HNC has been growing over the last several years. Published in 2016, a review article reported on 16 studies that looked at the role of physical activity and exercise in the patients with HNC[4] and found generally low activity rates of patients, with only 30.5% of patients meeting the physical activity guidelines before their cancer diagnosis in 1 study.[26] After treatment, these rates tend to be even lower if intervention is not offered. Rogers and colleagues[26] found that only 8.5% of cancer survivors were meeting physical activity guidelines at 1.5 years after treatment.

The fitness level of patients at the time of diagnosis must be considered in making medical decisions, such as types of treatments and appropriate interventions. The importance of physical activity and the education of patients on the value of increasing activity should be reinforced after diagnosis and throughout cancer treatments. After surgery and adjuvant therapy, maintaining a more active lifestyle may elicit better chances of recovery and improvement in physical and psychosocial functioning.[25,27–33] Although there are many potential barriers to increasing activity after diagnosis, such as dry mouth and throat, fatigue, drainage in the mouth or throat, eating difficulties, shortness of breath, muscle weakness, and swallowing difficulties, patients who increase their activity report improved symptom burden, decreased perceived barriers, and improved self-efficacy and control, thus reinforcing the value of discussion with patients.[34] Health care providers can play a key role in supporting and changing behaviors. A teachable moment for lifestyle change may present after a cancer diagnosis, during which health care providers can facilitate education and resources to support patients in reaching a more active lifestyle.[35,36]

Tailored Exercise as Therapy

Exercise, a subset of physical activity intended for specific health benefit, can be used for patients with HNC in the setting of rehabilitation. Members of this population face unique issues in rehabilitation, including deconditioning, weight loss, and fatigue.[9,37,38] This results largely from skeletal muscle wasting and cachexia, which may be related to the cancer itself, to treatment challenges, and to decreased activity. The size and extent of tumor at the primary site may result in impaired nutritional intake, contributing to weight loss and muscle wasting.[9] Full body resistance training plays an important role in preserving and rebuilding skeletal muscle and, therefore, a progressive resistance plan can help to optimize recovery outcomes in patients after treatment.[4]

Screening and assessment

The safety and efficacy of an exercise program is based on comprehensive patient screening, assessment and a tailored exercise prescription. Screening and assessment of patients is imperative before beginning a structured exercise program to ensure safety and improve the ability of tailoring an exercise prescription with the hopes of improving outcomes. Screening can include a general health questionnaire, the Physical Activity Readiness Questionnaire and questions specific to issues of most concern for individual patients with HNC (see **Table 1**). Screening to clear a patient for activity can be conducted by a physician or other medical practitioner, nurse practitioner, physiotherapist, or exercise specialist. Medical clearance, most often from the treating physician, is important before beginning an exercise program for those patients with active disease or those who are currently receiving treatment. Initial screening is intended to identify any factors that might risk the safety of a patient participating in a new exercise program. Specific recommendations and restrictions are helpful to guide the physiotherapist or exercise specialist in implementing the exercise program.

Once a patient has been screened and cleared, a physical therapist or exercise specialist can conduct a thorough assessment of the head, neck, and shoulder range of motion (ROM), strength, and sensory function, noting any pain or discomfort, deformity, or limitation. In addition, a full body assessment of overall aerobic fitness and general strength and flexibility should be conducted. Tests that are most clinically relevant and easy to administer may include a 6-minute walk test to assess aerobic functional status, hand grip dynamometer testing as an estimate of total upper body strength, and 30-second sit to stand test to determine lower body strength and endurance. With trained personnel and appropriate equipment, more in-depth assessment methods may be conducted, including aerobic or anaerobic cardiovascular testing on a stationary bike or treadmill, along with muscular strength and endurance testing using 1 or multiple repetition maximum testing, which has proven safe in members of this population.[39] An assessment of flexibility is very important,

especially in patients who have undergone surgery and may have decreased ROM contributing to chronic musculoskeletal issues. Goniometers and sit and reach devices can be helpful in assessing flexibility.

Prescription and tailoring

The previously discussed guidelines for physical activity (see **Box 1**), developed mainly from data in patients with breast, colorectal, and prostate cancer, provide effective guidelines for a broad range of patients. However, patients with HNC, often with significant skeletal muscle wasting and weight loss,[9] may demand a more targeted exercise program with the goal of increasing skeletal muscle mass and specific physical functional outcomes. Ideally, a tailored exercise rehabilitation program should increase overall activity while meeting or surpassing the general physical activity recommendations. Interventions of resistance training up to 30 ± 26 months after surgery, during adjuvant chemotherapy, or after adjuvant therapy, shows promise in mitigating muscle wasting and improving symptoms, such as tiredness, depression, anxiety, drowsiness, while improving overall well-being. The benefits have been found over the course of one fitness class and across a longitudinal 8- or 12-week program.[27,40] Structured exercise interventions typically include 6- to 12-week progressive resistance exercise programs, which generally involve 8 to 10 exercises, at approximately 70% to 85% of the patient's 1 repetition maximum, for 2 to 3 sets of approximately 6 to 12 repetitions.[4] This type of exercise program adheres to a hypertrophy prescription, progressing to an endurance prescription. An example of a full body resistance training program is shown in **Box 2**. Specific exercises of the program are based on individual needs, current limitations, and goals. Once an appropriate body weight is reached and maintained, moderate intensity aerobic type activity is introduced as warranted. Unfortunately, many patients treated for cancer are not counseled about specific whole body exercises that may help them to regain strength and function.

REHABILITATION FOR THE PATIENT WITH HEAD AND NECK CANCER
Physical Therapy

PT enhances, restores, and optimizes the function of musculoskeletal, neurologic, cardiorespiratory, and other systems. PT plays an active role in the symptom management of survivors of HNC focusing primarily on issues related to jaw, neck, and shoulder function that occur during or after

---

Box 2
Example exercise program for patients with head and neck cancer

Recommended prescription: 1 to 2 sets of 8 to 10 repetitions at 65% to 80% of 1 repetition maximum 1 to 2 days per week, progressing to 2 to 3 sets of 6 to 8 repetitions at 75% to 85% 1 repetition maximum 2 to 3 days per week. Choose 8 to 10 exercises per session.

This is a general example of a full-body strength training program. Modifications must be made to account for the unique needs and limitations of the individual patient. Patients may need to start with practicing exercise movements against gravity and then progress to low resistance, increasing accordingly. Avoid exacerbating neck or shoulder pathology.

Warm up: Light aerobic warm up for 5 to 10 minutes before starting strength training.

Upper body

- External shoulder rotation
- Internal shoulder rotation
- Lateral raise
- Anterior raise
- Shoulder press (provided there is no limitation for overhead movement)
- Chest press
- Row
- Lat pull down
- Bicep curls
- Triceps dips/extensions

Lower body

- Squat
- Forward lunge
- Lateral lunge
- Hamstring curl
- Knee extension

Core training

- Plank (progress from wall, to knees, to toes)
- Supine with knees at 90°, extend knees slightly and hold
- Bicycles (keep head and neck on supported pillow if neck pathology)
- Russian twists from seated

Flexibility: Finish with full body flexibility training, holding stretches for 30 to 60 seconds each. Spend extra time on neck and shoulder range of motion exercises.

---

treatment of cancer. Before beginning treatment for cancer, the focus of PT is to provide education on anticipated effects of cancer treatment and the planned course of rehabilitation. Ideally, evaluation of a patient before treatment informs of the baseline status and measurement of the following functions.

- Posture: resting position of head, presence of kyphosis.
- Jaw function and mouth opening (interincisor distance).
- Cervical spine active ROM.

- Shoulder active and passive ROM, scapular resting positioning and shoulder droop, and shoulder function.

After surgery

Early in the course after surgery, PT focuses on early mobilization (activity) and chest physiotherapy (ie, deep breathing, suctioning, positioning) to prevent postoperative complications.[41] Acute sequelae associated with surgical procedures include pain, sensory loss, neck and shoulder stiffness, and lymphedema. Patients with HNC who have undergone reconstruction with regional pedicled and free flaps require additional monitoring and precautions relating to reconstructive and tissue donor sites. Initially, restrictions after surgery related to neck and shoulder movements may be necessary to avoid excessive stress on the surgical incision and structures in the head and neck region. Observing these restrictions is especially important for patients who have undergone extensive neck dissection or those at risk of carotid blowout (**Table 3**).

Physical therapy treatment of the jaw and neck
PT programs have been shown to significantly improve treatment-related impairments owing to HNC in the jaw, neck, and shoulder regions[42,43] (see **Tables 1** and **2**).

Jaw Trismus, or limited mouth opening, is a known complication of oncologic treatments for HNC, including surgery and radiation therapy. Trismus is defined as an interincisal distance of less than 35 mm[6,9,20] and occurs in approximately one-third of survivors receiving cancer treatment in the region of oral cavity, oropharynx, nasopharynx, and temporomandibular joint.[7,21] Trismus may occur immediately after surgery, during radiation therapy, or present as a late effect occurring months after cancer treatment.[22] The impact of trismus on quality of life is profound, limiting key functions such as chewing, swallowing, and speech, as well as interfering with dental hygiene and dental management.[3–5] In the absence of interventions to prevent or attenuate development of trismus, the condition often becomes chronic and can be progressive in nature.[6]

Early intervention for trismus is considered key to reduce the risk of long-term morbidity. Multiple PT modalities are used in the treatment of trismus, with the most common including active exercises, manual therapy and use of a jaw opening devices such as the TheraBite Jaw Motion Rehabilitation[30] and the Dynasplint Trismus System.[31] Early evidence supports the benefit of preventative physiotherapy exercises with and without the use of assisted devices for improving interincisal distance during and after radiation therapy treatment. To address chronic trismus related to radiation fibrosis, significant benefit has been demonstrated with the introduction of assistive devices such as the Therabite and Dynasplint.[36–38]

Cervical spine Impairments related to the neck region include soft tissue restriction, muscle weakness, facial and neck lymphedema, and altered posture. Complications may occur owing to extensive surgical neck dissection procedures including removal of muscles such as the sternocleidomastoid. Moreover, even if preserved, in the case of the sternocleidomastoid muscle, function may be lost owing to damage to the blood supply to the muscle during the surgical procedure and/or as a result of an associated SAN injury.

Complications in the neck region from radiation therapy can occur months to years after treatment, and involve progressive fibrosis of the soft tissue in the anterior and lateral aspects of the neck. Active ROM exercises involving all planes of neck movement are initiated as soon as it is deemed safe after surgery. In survivors undergoing adjuvant radiation therapy, these exercises should be continued through radiation therapy if possible. In the event that the integrity of the skin and soft tissue of the neck region is compromised (eg, moist desquamation, blistering), exercises are withheld. Once the radiated skin has healed, ROM exercises should be recommenced and performed 2 to 3 times a day for a 6-month period or longer after radiation therapy, because repetition is of utmost importance. Although the exercises will not likely prevent the development of radiation-related tissue fibrosis, the goal of the exercises is to ensure the soft tissues of the neck heal in a lengthened rather than shortened position.

In the recovery stage after radiation therapy, stretching exercises can be introduced and survivors can be taught to provide an additional stretch to end-range lateral side flexion (side bending) and rotation by exerting gentle overpressure with the contralateral hand. Specific active stretches to the tissues in the anterior neck (eg, platysma and digastric muscles) are particularly helpful in addressing stiffness and edema in the region. Stretches should be held at the end range for 20 to 30 seconds and repeated between 4 and 6 times per session. If late presenting radiation fibrosis develops and is not responsive to a home exercise regimen approach, the therapist can introduce manual therapy and myofascial release techniques to help mobilize and lengthen the tissue.

Isometric strengthening exercises specific to the cervical deep flexors and extensors can start approximately 6 weeks after the completion of cancer treatment (surgery or radiation therapy). Postural correction using visual (mirrors) and manual cuing is often necessary for correct performance owing to diminished proprioception in the region. Survivors can benefit from technology (eg, phone reminders) or having family members remind them to correct posture.[44]

Lymphedema related to HNC is common after surgery but may also develop as a late effect of cancer treatment. Lymphedema commonly

Table 3
Physiotherapy interventions for head and neck cancer survivors

Timing	Procedure	Consequence/Effect	Physiotherapy Intervention	Focus/Comments
Immediate postoperatively	Surgery	Tracheostomy	Teaching for suctioning and chest physiotherapy to clear mucus and secretions from lungs	Prevention of postoperative complications
	Reconstruction	Deep vein thrombosis and pulmonary embolism	Early ambulation to promote circulation and keep lungs clear	Prevention of postoperative complications
		Flap site – reconstruction	Monitoring of healing	Avoid stress to healing tissues
		Fibular free flap	Gait retraining – use of mobility aid; weight-bearing restrictions in place	Keep leg elevated to attenuate swelling; High risk of developing trismus
~2 weeks postoperative (timing at discretion of surgeon)	Surgery with or without± neck dissection	Cervical spine pain and dysfunction	Cervical active ROM; edema management for face and neck	Caution – healing incision and tissues, and those undergoing extensive neck dissection or at risk of carotid blow out
		Postural dysfunction	Exercises to reinforce correct posture and proper breathing techniques	Reminders and cueing needed for posture
	Neck dissection	Shoulder dysfunction	Shoulder active ROM exercises	Focus on prevention of adhesive capsulitis
Prior/during radiation therapy	Oral or oropharyngeal surgery with or without reconstruction	TMJ dysfunction/trismus	Active exercises, manual mobilizations as indicated	Concern re: bone integrity if mandibulotomy or mandibular reconstruction with fibular flap
	Radiation therapy to neck region	Cervical: soft tissue contracture	Active ROM exercises; edema management for face and neck	Caution if acute tissue reaction to radiation therapy – limit ROM or stop exercises
	Neck dissection	Shoulder and scapular dysfunction	ROM exercises, stretching of pectoral muscle group; strengthening of compensatory muscles: emphasis on rhomboids, levator scapula	Avoid overhead activities, carrying or lifting heavy weights on side of surgery
Post cancer treatment	Surgery or radiation therapy	Trismus	Active exercises, manual therapy, provision of assistive device (eg, Therabite)	Attention to effects of radiation therapy, development of progressive tissue fibrosis
		Neck dysfunction	Active ROM and stretching exercises; manual therapy for radiation fibrosis; edema management for face and neck	Emphasis on ensuring healing of soft tissues in lengthened position for optimizing neck range and function
		Shoulder and scapular dysfunction	ROM exercises for shoulder; trapezius muscle activation and strengthening	Attention to status and recovery of spinal accessory nerve

Abbreviations: ROM, range of motion; TMJ, temporomandibular joint.

occurs in the face and neck region and tends to be worse in the morning and improve over the day as gravity assists with drainage of the region. Lymphedema management may include prescription of ROM exercises, manual lymph drainage, and self-massage to the region. Compression therapy is often helpful and can be applied with either off-the-shelf or custom-made garments. Kinesiotaping may be used to enhance drainage of the region in conjunction with other therapies, and is simple technique to apply, and comfortable for the survivor to wear. At present, there is currently a lack of research evidence examining neck dysfunction in the HNC population, with a single study, involving survivors with thyroid cancer, demonstrating benefit from active neck stretching exercises introduced on the first day after neck dissection surgery.[45]

Topic of interest: shoulder dysfunction

A common indication for referral to PT is to address shoulder pain and dysfunction related to resection or damage to the SAN.[46] The SAN, or cranial nerve XI, functions as a motor nerve for the trapezius and sternocleidomastoid muscles.[47] The SAN is vulnerable to injury from neck dissection involving the anterior or posterior cervical triangles.[39] Neurologic deficits associated with dissection include complete nerve lesions (neurotmesis), when the nerve is sacrificed or extensively damaged in a radical neck dissection, and incomplete nerve lesions (axonotmesis or neurapraxia), when the nerve is preserved intact.[39] Both complete and incomplete nerve lesions may present with similar shoulder dysfunction in the early postoperative period. With complete nerve lesions, full recovery of trapezius function is unlikely and ongoing shoulder syndrome ensues with pain, dysfunction, and permanent trapezius muscle denervation.[39] With nerve-sparing procedures, partial to full recovery of the nerve is expected within 18 months.[40] Owing to the lengthy recovery period, shoulder pain and dysfunction may develop secondary to malalignment of the scapula and shoulder complex.[39]

Shoulder impairments initially after neck dissection include pain, weakness, and limitation in active shoulder abduction movement.[39] Progressive atrophy of the trapezius muscle occurs over a 6- to 12-week period after surgery, resulting in a downward (depression) and forward (protraction) relocation of the resting position of scapula and shoulder complex, leading to shoulder droop.[44] On examination, there is visible change in the contour of the neck line, weakness in shoulder shrugging, "winging" of the medial border of

the scapula, and limitation in shoulder abduction to less than 90°.[44] Functionally, the impaired active ROM at the shoulder causes difficulty in simple overhead tasks such as washing hair, dressing, and reaching overhead. Secondarily, passive shoulder stiffness develops within a few weeks of surgery, unless passive and active-assisted ROM exercises are initiated.[44]

The course of SAN recovery after neck dissection surgery often varies even given similar neck dissections. For the purposes of PT intervention, SAN nerve recovery can be divided into 4 phases:

1. Acute phase: from 3 to 6 weeks postoperatively, the primary tissue healing phase;
2. Subacute phase: from 6 weeks to 3 to 6 months postoperatively, with no evidence of trapezius muscle activity and abduction ROM of less than 90°;
3. Nerve recovery phase: from 5 to 6 months postoperatively, with early signs of trapezius muscle recovery evident; and
4. Chronic phase: 18 months or more postoperatively, where the reinnervation potential of the SAN has peaked.

In the acute phase of SAN recovery and shoulder rehabilitation, the main principle of treatment is to protect the shoulder and maintain glenohumeral joint integrity. Although scapular dysfunction is anticipated after neck dissection, a secondary complication is adhesive capsulitis in the glenohumeral joint.[44] Once drains have been removed from the surgical site or after approval from the surgeon, gentle active ROM shoulder exercises are introduced to minimize pain and prevent stiffness of the shoulder postoperatively.[48] Providing education for proper positioning of the affected shoulder is paramount, such as supporting the shoulder and upper arm on pillows or armrests of a chair and preventing stretching of the weakened trapezius muscle.

In the subacute phase, PT treatment goals include maintaining shoulder passive ROM, preventing shoulder droop, eliminating pain, avoiding pectoralis muscle contracture, and improving scapular stabilization by strengthening alternative muscles to compensate for the functional loss of the trapezius muscle.[39] In this stage, owing to the malalignment of the scapula and weakness in the shoulder complex, completely avoiding overhead activities, pushing, pulling, and carrying activities involving heavy loads with the affected shoulder and arm is critical. For persistent pain, a shoulder orthosis may be prescribed to support the shoulder complex and minimize droop.[49]

In the nerve recovery phase, early signs of active trapezius muscle contraction will become evident in the upper portion of the trapezius muscle. Over the subsequent months, signs of middle and then lower trapezius muscle recovery are seen to improve scapular control and active abduction ROM. The focus of PT is on trapezius muscle reactivation and strengthening, including incorporating visual and manual cueing to help elicit proper trapezius muscle activation during exercises.[50] Over a 5- to 12-month period, as nerve and muscle further recover, shoulder pain most often resolves and a progressive increase in active shoulder elevation and abduction are observed.

In the chronic phase, once nerve function is restored or plateaus, PT intervention focuses on functional goals relating to leisure and productive activities. If nerve recovery is complete, compensation strategies may be discontinued and replaced with exercises to ensure proper scapulohumeral rhythm and to enhance trapezius muscle strength and power. For survivors with incomplete or no evidence of nerve recovery, compensation strategies may be continued permanently with activity adaptation to optimize function.

Current research supports PT treatment regimens ranging from ROM exercises to programs that include therapeutic exercise, manual therapy and the use of electrotherapeutic modalities.[48] Specific to survivors with SAN injury, progressive resistance exercise training has been shown to significantly reduce shoulder pain and disability, improve active ROM, and progress shoulder strength and endurance.[43]

Occupational Therapy

OT for patients with HNC focuses on maximizing function to achieve individualized goals.[51] OT models of practice target strengths and abilities, with interventions applied to functional participation, rather than to cure.[52] A successful intervention is gauged not necessarily by resolving the baseline issue, but by improving quality of life despite the issue. Enabling occupation includes everyday ADLs, such as dressing, feeding, and bathing, and more complex, instrumental ADLs such as driving, writing, working, or cooking. Referrals are indicated for patients with HNC who have short- or long-term issues requiring support to manage or improve current levels of function. Although interventions vary greatly, some OT interventions for members of the population are listed herein. Common complications and strategies are described in **Table 1**.

- Splinting: Addressing limited ROM, joint/bone/ muscle/ligament isolation, or progressive changes to typical movement patterns; for example, in a typical radial forearm free flap, splinting isolates the wrist but allows fingers to remain free.[51]
- Intervention for upper extremity function after oral reconstruction: Working closely with surgical teams after flap surgeries to ensure that, as flaps take to the oral cavity, the forearm area used as the donor source receives appropriate splinting, protective garments, and functional mobility interventions, to preserve hand dexterity and upper extremity function.[51]
- Lymphedema: Managing compression for edematous areas pretreatment and posttreatment (see **Table 1**).
- Cognitive function: Assessing and treating changes in thought patterns and processing, determining baseline cognition, and facilitating management of ADLs and instrumental ADLs.[51]
- Cancer-related fatigue management (see **Table 1**).

Topic of interest: return to work

Return to work is a significant issue impacting patients with HNC. In a metaanalysis of 36 articles investigating return to work across 21 countries, cancer survivors were twice as likely to be unemployed or disabled compared with a similar noncancer, working-age cohort at 33.8% compared with 15.2%, respectively.[53] Currently, access to cancer-specific, work-related rehabilitation is highly limited and not part of standard practice, despite emerging evidence that both prehabilitation and rehabilitation elicit positive outcomes for functional tasks.[54,55] The direct and secondary effects of HNC and associated treatments can have immediate and long-lasting physical and psychological challenges affecting function, in turn negatively impacting return to work. These challenges may include depleted energy through fatigue, sleep disturbance, and nutritional deficiencies; psychosocial issues, such as stress, anxiety, or depression; limited physical function through issues to joint mobility, decreased ROM, cervical myelopathy, trismus, and cervical dystonia; and decreased activity tolerance because of deconditioning.[55] Body image issues in patients with HNC are highly prevalent, potentially impact work functioning, and reduce confidence in communication.[55] Additionally, cognitive issues, commonly known as "brain fog," often present after cancer and related treatment, reducing the ability to complete complex work-related tasks, such as executive decision making and multitasking.[17] Issues surrounding typical workday tasks for both sedentary desk and more physical vocations present unique challenges in the development of return-to-work strategies in members of the HNC population.[11] A recent study of 66 working-aged HNC survivors found that participants who were not able to work reported lower quality of life scores, with more ongoing medical issues.[56]

Typical sedentary work, such as computer-related jobs, administrative or clerical roles, and driving tasks, primarily involves sitting and talking, reading, writing, typing, computer work, and multitasking. Managing complex hand tasks can be challenging for individuals with cervical neuropathy when they return to work; keyboards and work stations may require adaptation to facilitate dexterity and ease of communication. Further, depending on surgical and disease outcomes, a lack of saliva or changes to the anatomy of the mouth or jaw may make sustaining oral communication difficult. In these cases, typing may be more appropriate than speaking and referral to a speech-language pathologist may be recommended. For drivers, neck and shoulder ROM may be a barrier to returning to work. Such issues are highly challenging in patients with HNC and may exemplify some secondary complications likely to persist, often requiring a modification of vocational roles.[57] Without a thorough assessment of skills and abilities and without a specifically tailored yet flexible and adaptable return to work plan, a survivor of HNC survivor faces difficulty in reintegrating into the previous work role.

More physical vocations, such as trades work, mechanical-related jobs, and many health care and education roles, involve standing, balancing, bending, lifting, and moving. With deconditioning, neuropathy, and limited activity tolerance, survivors of HNC may face challenges managing fast-paced or physically difficult work environments. Upper extremity limitations may also impede an individual's ability to carry out physically challenging vocational tasks, warranting modified work plans or use of protective and supported braces or splints. Graduated or graded return to work plans prove more effective than directly returning to work.[58] Interdisciplinary collaboration among OT, PT, and exercise professionals to increase activity tolerance through functional exercise provides improvement in the length of time that an individual can tolerate task engagement. Focusing on the individual is a key component in the development of effective return to work interventions.

Across vocations, the impact of cancer-related fatigue and cognitive changes (brain fog) to HNC survivors can impede regular job functioning. In workplace environments, symptoms of fatigue and cognitive changes can be difficult to recognize, particularly with fatigue being common in the general population. Often the survivor and/or work team are not familiar with the distinction between cancer-related fatigue and cognitive changes as compared with typical fatigue and cognitive issues.[59] Given that cancer-related fatigue and cognitive changes are known to vary and fluctuate in presentation, research suggests that self-report is a key method of determining an individual's duration of activity tolerance and thus the appropriate number of complex or multistep tasks that an individual can manage.[60] Although cognitive issues often abate in the months after treatment, fatigue can last years after treatment.[17,59] The engagement in early education can elicit beneficial long-term results for survivors in the management of fatigue and cognitive changes.[58] The positive impact of physical activity on fatigue and cognition suggest that individuals who engage in mobility-related tasks eventually improve work-related activity.[61]

The past expectation that cancer survivors will return to work after treatment without issue is currently proven a fallacy. Studies suggest that a successful, return to work interventions must focus on individualized goals and barriers to function, using a specific work-related series of targeted goals over a specified period of time.[62] Evidence shows that (1) positive productive work environments can lead to perceived improvements in wellness and (2) individuals may use coping skills and change behaviors as a means to participate in meaningful activities.[56] Qualitative research indicates that individuals who feel supported in their work, home, and medical environments tend to fare better in the transition to work after illness than do those who are stressed or feel unsupported.[63] Understanding how patients with HNC address work-related transitions will support future intervention and develop protocols of managing vocational rehabilitation. Future research must consider targeted vocational interventions, physical and functional activity guidelines for workplaces, and functions-based pilot programming for return to work tailored to members of the HNC population.

SUMMARY

Currently, increasing rates of HNC incidence and survival after treatment are demanding rehabilitation interventions that maximize function and recovery after a diagnosis and cancer treatment. Evidence supports the role for physical activity, exercise, PT and OT as important components of a rehabilitation program to aid symptom management and functional recovery while improving quality of life. The American Cancer Society's Survivorship Recommendations suggest all patients with HNC should be assessed for rehabilitation, because the early identification of impairments and functional limitations, both during and after cancer treatment, are clearly essential for timely physical rehabilitation and OT interventions.

REFERENCES

1. Argiris A, Karamouzis MV, Raben D, et al. Head and neck cancer. Lancet 2008;371(9625):1695–709.
2. Haddad RI, Shin DM. Recent advances in head and neck cancer. N Engl J Med 2008;359(11):1143–54.
3. Lango MN. Multimodal treatment for head and neck cancer. Surg Clin North Am 2009;89(1):43–52, viii.
4. Capozzi LC, Nishimura KC, McNeely ML, et al. The Impact of physical activity on health related fitness and quality of life for head and neck cancer patients: a systematic review. Br J Sports Med 2016;50(6): 325–38.
5. Marur S, D'Souza G, Westra WH, et al. HPV-associated head and neck cancer: a virus-related cancer epidemic. Lancet Oncol 2010;11(8):781–9.
6. Cohen EE, LaMonte SJ, Erb NL, et al. American cancer society head and neck cancer survivorship care guideline. CA Cancer J Clin 2016;66(3):203–39.
7. Schmitz KH, Courneya KS, Matthews C, et al. American College of Sports Medicine roundtable on exercise guidelines for cancer survivors. Med Sci Sports Exerc 2010;42(7):1409–26.
8. Rock CL, Doyle C, Demark-Wahnefried W, et al. Nutrition and physical activity guidelines for cancer survivors. CA Cancer J Clin 2012;62(4):243–74.
9. Silver HJ, Dietrich MS, Murphy BA. Changes in body mass, energy balance, physical function, and inflammatory state in patients with locally advanced head and neck cancer treated with concurrent chemoradiation after low-dose induction chemotherapy. Head Neck 2007;29(10):893–900.
10. Stout NL, Levy E, Pfalzer L. Upper quadrant impairments associated with cancer treatment. Top Geriatr Rehabil 2011;27(3):222–33.
11. Pergolotti M, Williams GR, Campbell C, et al. Occupational therapy for adults with cancer: why it matters. Oncologist 2016;21(3):314–9.
12. Bang MS, Lee S. Musculoskeletal disorders, pain and rehabilitation. 3rd edition. Philadelphia: Elsevier Saunders; 2015.
13. Trombly Latham C. Occupational Therapy for Physical Dysfunction. 6th edition. Baltimore (MD): Wolters Kluwer; Lippincott Williams & Wilkins; 2008.
14. Sherman AC, Simonton S, Adams DC, et al. Coping with head and neck cancer during different phases of treatment. Head Neck 2000;22(8):787–93.
15. Bensadoun RJ, Riesenbeck D, Lockhart PB, et al. A systematic review of trismus induced by cancer therapies in head and neck cancer patients. Support Care Cancer 2010;18(8):1033–8.
16. Al Niaimi F, Cox N. Cellulitis and lymphoedema: a vicious cycle. J Lymphoedema 2009;4(2):38–42.
17. Silver JK, Gilchrist LS. Cancer rehabilitation with a focus on evidence-based outpatient physical and occupational therapy interventions. Am J Phys Med Rehabil 2011;90(5):S5–15.
18. Barber B, Dergousoff J, Slater L, et al. Depression and survival in patients with head and neck cancer: a systematic review. JAMA Otolaryngol Head Neck Surg 2016;142(3):284–8.
19. Langius JA, van Dijk AM, Doornaert P, et al. More than 10% weight loss in head and neck cancer patients during radiotherapy is independently associated with deterioration in quality of life. Nutr Cancer 2013;65(1):76–83.
20. Caspersen CJ, Powell KE, Christenson GM. Physical activity, exercise, and physical fitness: definitions and distinctions for health-related research. Public Health Rep 1985;100(2):126–31.
21. Speck RM, Courneya KS, Masse LC, et al. An update of controlled physical activity trials in cancer survivors: a systematic review and meta-analysis. J Cancer Surviv 2010;4(2):87–100.
22. Ballard-Barbash R, Friedenreich CM, Courneya KS, et al. Physical activity, biomarkers, and disease outcomes in cancer survivors: a systematic review. J Natl Cancer Inst 2012;104(11):815–40.
23. Fong DY, Ho JW, Hui BP, et al. Physical activity for cancer survivors: meta-analysis of randomised controlled trials. BMJ 2012;344:e70.
24. Thijs KM, de Boer AG, Vreugdenhil G, et al. Rehabilitation using high-intensity physical training and long-term return-to-work in cancer survivors. J Occup Rehabil 2012;22(2):220–9.
25. Samuel SR, Arun Maiya G, Babu AS, et al. Effect of exercise training on functional capacity & quality of life in head & neck cancer patients receiving chemoradiotherapy. Indian J Med Res 2013; 137(3):515–20.
26. Rogers LQ, Courneya KS, Robbins KT, et al. Physical activity and quality of life in head and neck cancer survivors. Support Care Cancer 2006;14(10): 1012–9.
27. Capozzi LC, Boldt KR, Lau H, et al. A clinic-supported group exercise program for head and neck cancer survivors: managing cancer and treatment side effects to improve quality of life. Support Care Cancer 2015;23(4):1001–7.
28. Lonbro S, Dalgas U, Primdahl H, et al. Feasibility and efficacy of progressive resistance training and dietary supplements in radiotherapy treated head and neck cancer patients-the DAHANCA 25A study. Acta Oncol 2013;52(2):310–8.

29. Lonbro S, Dalgas U, Primdahl H, et al. Lean body mass and muscle function in head and neck cancer patients and healthy individuals–results from the DAHANCA 25 study. Acta Oncol 2013;52(7):1543–51.

30. Eades M, Murphy J, Carney S, et al. Effect of an interdisciplinary rehabilitation program on quality of life in patients with head and neck cancer: review of clinical experience. Head Neck 2013; 35(3):343–9.

31. Rogers LQ, Anton PM, Fogleman A, et al. Pilot, randomized trial of resistance exercise during radiation therapy for head and neck cancer. Head Neck 2013; 35(8):1178–88.

32. Aghili M, Farhan F, Rade M. A pilot study of the effects of programmed aerobic exercise on the severity of fatigue in cancer patients during external radiotherapy. Eur J Oncol Nurs 2007;11(2):179–82.

33. Crevenna R, Schneider B, Mittermaier C, et al. Implementation of the Vienna Hydrotherapy Group for Laryngectomees–a pilot study. Support Care Cancer 2003;11(11):735–8.

34. Rogers LQ, Courneya KS, Robbins KT, et al. Physical activity correlates and barriers in head and neck cancer patients. Support Care Cancer 2008; 16(1):19–27.

35. Jones LW, Courneya KS, Fairey AS, et al. Effects of an oncologist's recommendation to exercise on self-reported exercise behavior in newly diagnosed breast cancer survivors: a single-blind, randomized controlled trial. Ann Behav Med 2004;28(2): 105–13.

36. Demark-Wahnefried W, Aziz NM, Rowland JH, et al. Riding the crest of the teachable moment: promoting long-term health after the diagnosis of cancer. J Clin Oncol 2005;23(24):5814–30.

37. Couch M, Lai V, Cannon T, et al. Cancer cachexia syndrome in head and neck cancer patients: part I. Diagnosis, impact on quality of life and survival, and treatment. Head Neck 2007;29(4):401–11.

38. Couch ME, Dittus K, Toth MJ, et al. Cancer cachexia update in head and neck cancer: definitions and diagnostic features. Head Neck 2015; 37(4):594–604.

39. McNeely ML, Parliament M, Courneya KS, et al. A pilot study of a randomized controlled trial to evaluate the effects of progressive resistance exercise training on shoulder dysfunction caused by spinal accessory neurapraxia/neurectomy in head and neck cancer survivors. Head Neck 2004;26(6): 518–30.

40. Sandmael JA, Bye A, Solheim TS, et al. Feasibility and preliminary effects of resistance training and nutritional supplements during versus after radiotherapy in patients with head and neck cancer: a pilot randomized trial. Cancer 2017;123(22):4440–8.

41. Packel L. Oncological diseases and disorders. In: Malone DJ, Bishop Lindsay KL, editors. Physical therapy in acute care: a clinician's guide. Thorofare (NJ): Slack Incorporated; 2006. p. 503–44.

42. Dijkstra PU, Sterken MW, Pater R, et al. Exercise therapy for trismus in head and neck cancer. Oral Oncol 2007;43(4):389–94.

43. Carvalho AP, Vital FM, Soares BG. Exercise interventions for shoulder dysfunction in patients treated for head and neck cancer. Cochrane Database Syst Rev 2012;(4):CD008693.

44. Patten C, Hillel AD. The 11th nerve syndrome. Accessory nerve palsy or adhesive capsulitis? Arch Otolaryngol Head Neck Surg 1993;119(2):215–20.

45. Takamura Y, Miyauchi A, Tomoda C, et al. Stretching exercises to reduce symptoms of postoperative neck discomfort after thyroid surgery: prospective randomized study. World J Surg 2005;29(6):775–9.

46. Medina J. Neck dissection. In: Bailey BJ, editor. Head and neck surgery- otolaryngology. 4th edition. Philadelphia: Lippincott Williams and Wilkins; 2006. p. 1595–610.

47. Fehrenbach MJ, Herring SW. Illustrated anatomy of the head and neck. 2nd edition. Philadelphia: W.B. Saunders; 2002.

48. Tuohy SM, Savodnik A. Postsurgical rehabilitation in cancer. In: Stubblefield MD, O'Dell MW, editors. Cancer rehabilitation: principles and practice. New York: Demos Medical; 2009. p. 813–24.

49. Kizilay A, Kalcioglu MT, Saydam L, et al. A new shoulder orthosis for paralysis of the trapezius muscle after radical neck dissection: a preliminary report. Eur Arch Otorhinolaryngol 2006;263(5): 477–80.

50. McNeely ML, Parliament MB, Seikaly H, et al. Effect of exercise on upper extremity pain and dysfunction in head and neck cancer survivors: a randomized controlled trial. Cancer 2008;113(1):214–22.

51. Elizabeth BGT. Enabling occupation: an occupational therapy perspective. Ontario (Canada): Canadian Association of Occupational Therapists; 2002.

52. Turpin M, Iwama M. Using occupational therapy models in practice. Edinburgh (United Kingdom): Churchill Livingstone Elsevier; 2011.

53. Groeneveld IF, de Boer AGEM, Frings-Dresen MHW. Physical exercise and return to work: cancer survivors' experiences. J Cancer Surviv 2013;7(2): 237–46.

54. Silver JK, Baima J. Cancer prehabilitation: an opportunity to decrease treatment-related morbidity, increase cancer treatment options, and improve physical and psychological health outcomes. Am J Phys Med Rehabil 2013;92(8):715–27.

55. Jacobson JJ, Epstein JB, Eichmiller FC, et al. The cost burden of oral, oral pharyngeal, and salivary gland cancers in three groups: commercial insurance, Medicare, and Medicaid. Head Neck Oncol 2012;4(1):15.

56. Isaksson J, Wilms T, Laurell G, et al. Meaning of work and the process of returning after head and neck cancer. Support Care Cancer 2016;24(1):205–13.

57. Yuen HK, Gillespie MB, Day TA, et al. Driving behaviors in patients with head and neck cancer during and after cancer treatment: a preliminary report. Head Neck 2007;29(7):675–81.

58. Cooper AF, Hankins M, Rixon L, et al. Distinct work-related, clinical and psychological factors predict return to work following treatment in four different cancer types. Psychooncology 2013;22(3):659–67.

59. Wefel JS, Schagen SB. Chemotherapy-related cognitive dysfunction. Curr Neurol Neurosci Rep 2012;12(3):267–75.

60. Sherman AC, Simonton S. Advances in quality of life research among head and neck cancer patients. Curr Oncol Rep 2010;12(3):208–15.

61. de Boer AGEM, Taskila TK, Tamminga SJ, et al. Interventions to enhance return-to-work for cancer patients. Cochrane Database of Systematic Review 2011;2:CD007569.

62. Pearce A, Timmons A, O'Sullivan E, et al. Long-term workforce participation patterns following head and neck cancer. J Cancer Surviv 2015;9(1):30–9.

63. Dewa CS, Trojanowski L, Tamminga SJ, et al. Work-related experiences of head and neck cancer survivors: an exploratory and descriptive qualitative study. Disabil Rehabil 2018;40(11):1252–8.

Maxillofacial Prosthetics

Kamolphob Phasuk, DDS, MS*, Steven P. Haug, DDS, MSD

KEYWORDS

- Maxillofacial prosthetics • Maxillofacial prosthodontics • Obturator prosthesis
- Head and neck neoplasms—rehabilitation • Facial prosthesis

KEY POINTS

- Maxillofacial prosthetics is a branch of prosthodontics associated with restoration and/or replacement of stomatognathic and craniofacial structure with prostheses, which may or may not be removed on a regular or elective basis.
- After cancer ablation surgery in the head and neck region, a maxillofacial prosthesis can rehabilitate a patient's appearance and functions, including mastication, swallowing, and speech.
- When surgical construction after cancer ablation surgery is limited, patient functioning and esthetics can be restored by a maxillofacial prosthesis. Patient quality of life and psychological status are improved.
- A maxillofacial prosthodontist works closely with the oncologic surgeon, physicians, and others cancer care team members to deliver the best treatment outcome for the patient.

INTRODUCTION

Maxillofacial prosthetics is a branch of prosthodontics associated with restoration and/or replacement of stomatognathic and craniofacial structures with prostheses, which may or may not be removed on a regular or elective basis.[1] After cancer ablation surgery in the head and neck region, a maxillofacial prosthesis can rehabilitate a patient's appearance and functioning, including mastication, swallowing, and speech. Not just after surgical treatment, but on many other occasions the maxillofacial prosthodontist is requested to fabricate a device to support the ongoing cancer treatment. A positioned radiation stent for radiation therapy and a feeding appliance are good examples of those devices. In general, a maxillofacial prosthodontist works closely with the oncologic surgeon, physicians, and others cancer care team members to deliver the best treatment outcome for the patient.

PROSTHETICS MANAGEMENT OF PATIENT AFTER MAXILLARY RESECTION SURGERY

Surgical excision of tumors in the maxilla is a principle reason for a maxillectomy or a maxillary resection surgery.[2,3] Even though it depends on the type and location of the tumor, cancer ablation surgery of the maxilla often involves hard palate, maxillary sinus, and nasal cavity. An alteration of the hard palate as the result of surgery can create a communication between the oral cavity and the nasal cavity. Because of this oronasal communication, a food bolus and liquids can escape the oral cavity to exit the nares. The failure to impound the air causes a sound distortion called hypernasality. The consequences of a maxillary defect can lead to unintelligible speech and difficulty eating with a potential for inadequate nutrition intake. Prosthetic intervention, with a maxillary obturator prosthesis, is necessary to restore the contour of the hard palate and to recreate the functional separation of the oral cavity and nasal

Disclosure Statement: The authors have nothing to disclose.
Department of Prosthodontics, Indiana University School of Dentistry, 1121 West Michigan Street, Indianapolis, IN 46202, USA
* Corresponding author.
E-mail address: kphasuk@iu.edu

Oral Maxillofacial Surg Clin N Am 30 (2018) 487–497
https://doi.org/10.1016/j.coms.2018.06.009
1042-3699/18/© 2018 Elsevier Inc. All rights reserved.

cavity and maxillary sinus.[4] This prosthetic intervention can be started as early as at the time of the maxillary resection surgery and will be necessary for the remainder of the patient's life.

PROSTHETIC TREATMENT PLANNING

Treatment planning of prosthodontic rehabilitation for the patient undergoing maxillary resection surgery starts before the surgery. The principle when treating maxillectomy patients preoperatively is a comprehensive evaluation, in a limited time, to maximize the health status after surgery and maintain the usefulness of the remaining teeth.[2,3] A comprehensive oral and dental examination should be performed and dental radiographs should be taken. An accurate study cast that includes all important anatomy has to be obtained (**Fig. 1**) and mounted in an appropriate articulator.[5] It is preferred to have at least 2 sets of casts. One is preserved as a pretreatment record and other may be used to fabricate the surgical obturator or interim obturator. Irreversible hydrocolloid is generally the material of choice for making the impression for study casts. This material has an innate property that captures anatomic details in a short clinical working time and is gentle to soft tissue, which is especially important around a tumor. When possible, dental prophylaxis or gross debridement should be performed as well as any minor operative dental procedures. These dental preventative measures minimize the risk of dental and periodontal problems owing to the difficulty of oral hygiene practice postoperatively. Unsalvageable teeth should also be removed at the time of surgery or preoperatively.

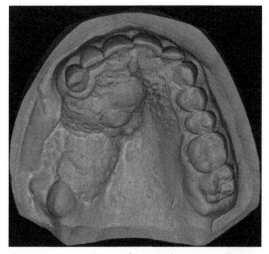

Fig. 1. Preoperative study cast for a maxilletomy patient.

It is very important to discuss with the patient the plan for oral rehabilitation. Most patients are not familiar with the services that the prosthodontist can provide. The benefits, limitations, and sequence of the prosthodontic treatment plan should be explained to the patients and their family. Patient compliance and acceptance are very important for the success of the treatment.

Prosthetics rehabilitation for maxillary resection surgery can be classified into 3 phases[4,5]:

- Surgical/immediate obturation,
- Postoperative/interim obturation, and
- Definitive obturation.

Surgical/Immediate Obturation

Surgical obturation has many benefits for the either edentulous or dental patients who require any type of maxillectomy or palatalectomy. The benefits of surgical obturation include providing a matrix on which the surgical packing can be placed and a decrease in the risk of oral contamination to the wound. The prosthesis improves the patient's psychological status by enabling the patient to speak and swallow immediately after surgery. The ability to swallow immediately after surgery may eliminate the need for a nasogastric tube or facilitate earlier removal. When using a surgical obturator, the hospitalization period potentially reduces to 3 to 5 days after surgery.[5]

Communication between the prosthodontist and the surgeon is critical for the design and fabrication of the surgical obturator prosthesis. The goal of a head and neck surgeon is to achieve complete oncologic resection of the tumor and leave clear margins at the resected site. However, for prosthodontic rehabilitation after maxillary resection surgery, maintaining as many structures (eg, hard palate, teeth) as possible is the key to improving functional outcomes with a maxillary obturator. In general, the prognosis of the prosthodontic rehabilitation of edentulous patient varies with the defect size.[6] For the dentate patient, the more alveolar process and teeth that are preserved, the better the functional outcome of the prosthesis. The surgical incision line also greatly influences the design and extension of the surgical obturator. One should design an obturator with the most conservative line of resection. By using the most conservative surgical planning, the prosthesis may be used even if the defect is larger than previously planned. However, if the most extensive line of resection is used for design and less tissue is resected at the time of surgery, the surgical obturator could be too large and would require an adjustment in the operating room. In some institutions, maxillofacial prosthodontists are part of the operative team and can make necessary intraoperative adjustments. However, prosthodontists are not always in the operating room and, thus, preoperative communication is critical between the head and neck ablative surgeon and the prosthodontist. This communication of surgical extent ensures appropriate sizing and fit of the temporary surgical obturator for the maximum postoperative benefit.

When considering the extent of surgical resection, the head and neck surgeon and prosthodontist should discuss performing maxillectomy through the socket of an extracted tooth rather than at the interproximal area.[6] An interproximal cut will result in resorption of the alveolar bone of the remaining teeth adjacent to the defect. This factor will eventually compromise periodontal health and vitality of the tooth next to the defect, which may likely lead to the loss of tooth. The tooth adjacent to the defect is an important abutment for the obturator prosthesis. If possible, the alveolar process that supports the tooth should be maintained.

There are several considerations for fabricating the surgical obturator. The surgical obturator should have a simple design, and be lightweight and inexpensive.[5] A clear heat processed acrylic resin or autopolymerizing acrylic resin is the material of choice for fabricating a surgical obturator.[4] The benefit of a clear acrylic resin is the ability to visualize the underlying tissue at the time of placement in the operating room and during the early healing period. For the edentulous patient, a peripheral extension should be made to the proper extension of a complete denture without overextension. Approximating the extension of the prosthesis into the soft palate and the pterygoid plate, especially in an edentulous patient, should be avoided. At the surgical defect or the skin graft–mucosa junction, the extension of the prosthesis should be terminated slightly short. The surgical packing will close any discrepancies between the surgical defect margin and the margin of the surgical obturator.[4]

The surgical obturator prosthesis for a dentate patient should be perforated at the interproximal area to allow the prosthesis to be secured with wire to the teeth at the time of surgery (**Fig. 2**). Securing the surgical obturator prosthesis for the edentulous patient is more challenging. It requires the use of a palatal bone screw. A titanium or stainless steel bone screw can be placed through the predrilled holes of the prosthesis at the anterior peak of palatal vault into the vomer. If the vomer is resected, 2 screws can be placed through the prosthesis into the lateral hard palate at the conflicting angle.[4]

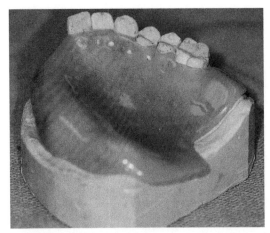

Fig. 2. Processed surgical obturator with perforated holes ready for the surgery.

In general, the original palatal contour should be reproduced. Anterior teeth can be included in the surgical obturator for psychological and speech reasons. However, posterior occlusion should be avoided to minimize the risk of trauma to the surgical defect area.

Postoperative/Interim Obturation

After the initial healing period, approximately 7 to 10 days postoperatively, the surgical obturator prosthesis and surgical packing are removed. A definitive prosthesis is not indicated until the surgical site is healed and dimensionally stable.[5] The complete healing time for the surgical site may be up to 3 to 4 months or more if radiation is included in the regimen. In this period, the interim obturator prosthesis is needed to restore function, such as speech and swallowing, as well as esthetics for the patient. The interim obturator also helps to improve the patient's psychological and emotional status.

For the completely edentulous patient, the prosthesis base used for surgical obturator can be modified to serve as an interim obturator prosthesis. The base plate is border molded and relined using soft liner material (prosthesis polyethyl methacrylates acrylic resins; **Fig. 3**). The viscosity of the material can be altered by changing ratio of powder (polymer) and liquid (monomer). This material also has great handling properties and can be shaped manually.[4] The residual hard palate area and border area should be relined first for optimum stability of the base plate. The defect area can be impressed starting from the bony tissue border. The periphery of the of the defect is impressed by manually and arbitrary extending the soft liner material and then adding the material incrementally. During impression of the defect site, the patient

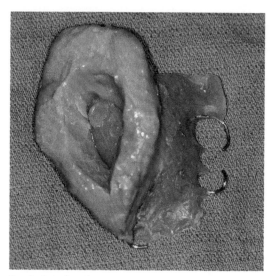

Fig. 3. Interim obturator.

should be directed to perform exaggerated head movements and swallowing motions. This technique is an attempt to simulate a functional movement and should be performed with any addition of incremental of soft liner material. After this functional impression, the base plate with impression material is flasked and processed with autopolymerizing or heat polymerizing acrylic resin and delivered to the patient within a few hours.

The simple ways to evaluate the performance of the obturator are by speech and swallowing.[7] The only speech sounds in English that are formed when air passes through the nasal cavity are 'n', 'm', and 'ng'. Some authors have suggested to listen to patient recreate the 'm' sound and the 'b' sound.[4] If the 'b' is clear and distinct, then there is no air escaping beyond the obturator. The phenomenon of air escape from the oral cavity to the nasal cavity during speech is called hypernasal speech. Another method to evaluate the obturator prosthesis is by drinking water. With the prosthesis in place, the patient should be able to drink water without nasal leakage in an upright position.

The same general principles apply to the dentate patient. However, the interim prosthesis or prosthesis base should be fabricated from a duplication of the second set of casts. This acrylic resin base should incorporate retentive wires in strategic locations. Soft liner material can also be used to reline and make a functional impression of the defect site. Patients should be educated that, throughout the healing period, an interim prosthesis needs to be routinely revised to maintain the performance of prosthesis. Once the defect site is stable, the prosthetics rehabilitation process should continue to definitive obturation.

If the opposing mandibular teeth are present, having a single posterior occlusal contact position increases the stability of the prosthesis. Home care instructions should also be given to the patient in this phase including dental hygiene, defect cleaning, and prosthesis care.

Definitive Obturation

During the healing period, patients should see their prosthodontist every 2 to 3 weeks for any needed revisions of the interim prosthesis. By 3 to 4 months, most patients have adjusted mentally and have realized that their mastication and speech will not be substantially compromised. It may be several months after surgery before the surgical area is completely stable without tissue change. This may be up to 6 to 12 months after completion of therapy depending on the size of the defect site.[4,5] Also, healing time may be affected by the radiation treatment. In the late interim phase before the definitive obturation, any auxiliary treatments such as endodontic and periodontic work should be completed. Additionally, all the remaining teeth should be reevaluated. Preliminary impressions are made and study casts are properly mounted. The prosthodontics rehabilitation plan should be developed systematically and thoroughly owing to the multiple considerations, which differ from a routine prosthodontic patient. Movement of the prosthesis will be significant during functioning.

For the edentulous patient, without an osseointegrated dental implant, it is very difficult for a prosthesis to stay in place without using denture adhesive. Indeed, collaboration and involvement of an oral maxillofacial surgeon from the initial planning of the oral prosthesis is important. Placement of an osseointegrated dental implant can significantly improve the function of obturator prosthesis.[5] Suitable locations for osseointegrated dental implants include the anterior maxilla and the maxillary tuberosity.[5,8] The osseointegrated dental implant placement can be done at the time of surgery or at some appropriate time thereafter. Radiation is a critical factor that could compromise the short-term and long-term osseous integration and durability of dental implants in this patient population.[8,9] The patient's quality of life, prosthesis performance, risks, and benefits are factors to consider for using an osseointegrated dental implant to support and stabilize the obturator prosthesis. However, with or without an additional support from the dental implant, the principle is to preserve the hard palate, residual ridge, and healthy abutment teeth for the maximum support, stability, and retention of the prosthesis (**Fig. 4**).

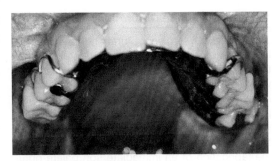

Fig. 4. Definitive obturator.

COMBINED SURGICAL-PROSTHETIC REHABILITATION

Recent advances in computed tomography imaging and medical modeling have facilitated preplanning for complex surgical reconstruction of the mandible and the maxilla using vascularized free flaps. This advancement also facilitates prosthodontic rehabilitation of the oral cavity for both functional and cosmetic purposes. Indeed, implant supported prostheses can be used to effectively restore function and esthetics for the patient.[5,10] This planning is often most desirable in a younger patient population that is healthier, but it can be applied to wide range of patients. The patient selection for this combined surgical and prosthetic rehabilitation is very important. The defect site must be proven to be free of disease and sufficient (>2 cm) in size.[5] The common donor sites used for bone reconstruction are iliac crest, scapular, and especially fibula free flaps.[10] Careful prosthetic and surgical planning are required. Computer software using computed tomography data is used to create a 3-dimensional model with fabrication technology (eg, a stereolithography model). The oral maxillofacial surgeon, head and neck surgeon, and the prosthodontist can then collaborate over this model to identify ideal locations for the reconstruction, the osseointegrated dental implants, the titanium plate, and the subsequent prosthesis. Osseointegrated dental implants can be placed simultaneously in the free vascularized graft at the time of surgery (1-stage procedure). However, malangulation of the dental implants and compromise of flap vascularization are risks of a 1-stage approach. As a result of these risks, many institutions prefer a 2-stage surgical approach. This technique allows 6 to 12 months of healing and vascularization of the free fibular graft. Osseointegrated dental implants are then placed after radiation and healing is complete. Prosthetic rehabilitation will start 4 to 6 months later for an adequate time of healing and osseointegration of the dental implant.

Prosthetics reconstruction of the dentate patient with reasonable remaining teeth and hard palate can be achieved by a removable partial denture obturator prosthesis. Normal speech and swallowing can be restored as well as reasonable mastication. Creating a favorable defect (eg, skin graft of the defect, conservative incision line to preserve healthy periodontal structures of key abutments) for the prosthesis is the key to success of the rehabilitation. This process requires good communication and collaboration with the oncologic surgeon and maxillofacial prosthodontist before the tumor ablation surgery. For the edentulous patient, speech and swallowing can be restored but mastication remains a challenge (**Fig. 5**). Using dental implants in the residual ridge significantly improves the performance of the prosthesis, especially during mastication.

Finally, home care and oral hygiene are very important to long-term success and satisfaction. Irrigation of the defect daily with normal saline is recommended. The removable prosthesis should not be kept outside of the mouth for an extended period of time. The prosthesis should also be in place after cleaning with each meal. Daily teeth and implant cleaning with proper modalities needs to be reinforced to the patient to maintain the health of the remaining oral tissue.

PROSTHETIC MANAGEMENT OF THE SOFT PALATE DEFECT

The soft palate is a complex neuromuscular aponeurosis.[11] It consists of multiple muscles such as the tensor veli palateni, the palatoglossus, the palatopharyngeus, the levator veli palateni, and the musculus uvula muscles.[12] These muscles are innervated by the pharyngeal plexus (vagus nerve, cranial nerve X), except for the tensor veli palatine, which is innervated by mandibular division of trigeminal cranial nerve (cranial nerve V). The physiologic function in this

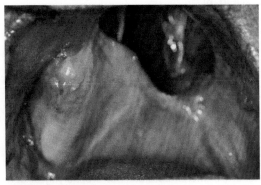

Fig. 5. Maxillary defect (edentulous).

region, also known as a velopharyngeal function, requires a simultaneous movement of the muscles in this area.[13,14] One or a combination of structural and motor limitations within the velopharyngeal mechanism can result in velopharyngeal dysfunction. This velopharyngeal dysfunction can result in hypernasality and poor intelligibility of speech.[13,15] In general, there are 2 terms that are used to describe velopharyngeal dysfunction based on physical and/or structural integrity. Palatopharyngeal/velopharyngeal insufficiency describes velopharyngeal dysfunction when there is a tissue or structural defect of the velum or pharyngeal wall resulting in unaccomplished closure at the level of the nasopharynx.[11,16] When the soft palate and the pharyngeal structures are of adequate dimension but fail to close the nasopharynx because of muscular and/or neurologic incapacity, the term palatopharyngeal/velopharyngeal incompetency applies.[11]

Surgical excision of neoplastic disease in the soft palate area can include the soft palate and adjacent structures.[13,17] The delicate functional balance between muscles and the velopharyngeal mechanism is often affected by surgery, but the degree of this dysfunction depends on the extent of surgical resection and method of surgical closure.[13] When the function of the palatopharyngeal area is altered owing to the insufficient structures after the tumor resection, an obturator prosthesis can be designed to close the opening between residual soft palate and the pharynx.[11] The goals of the pharyngeal obturator prosthesis, also known as speech bulb prosthesis or speech aid prosthesis, are to provide an adequate ability to control nasal emission during speech and to prevent the leakage of material into the nasal passage during swallowing.[5,14,18,19] Similar to a hard palate defect, prosthetic treatment for the acquired soft palate defect patient can be approached as immediate/surgical obturation, interim/delayed obturation, and definitive obturation (**Fig. 6**).

Surgical/Immediate Obturation

The immediate/surgical obturation is most useful in the dentate or partially edentulous patient.[14,18,19] In the edentulous patient or the patient with limited medial or lateral posterior border resection, a delayed obturation approach is preferred.[19] The immediate obturator prosthesis will additionally provide support and retention of the surgical packing. The greatest challenge in the fabrication of an immediate soft palate obturator prosthesis is a proper soft palate extension. For example, the drape of the intact soft palate precludes the clinician from obtaining an impression of the nasopharynx in which normal palatopharyngeal closure occurs[5,19] Also, it is very difficult to delineate the surgical margins before the operation. Adjustments at surgery are generally required for the proper extension without excessive tissue contact as well as providing space for a nasogastric tube.

Postoperative/Interim Obturation

At 7 to 10 days after the surgery, the prosthesis and surgical pack are removed. The tissue contact, especially at the lateral and posterior border, are checked. Then the soft liner material is used to correct the palatopharyngeal extension area of the prosthesis. The patient is instructed to perform head movements and swallowing movements to mold the extension area to the proper dimension.[19] Speech and swallowing are evaluated. The patient is followed with sequential appointments until a definitive prosthesis can be fabricated.

Definitive Obturation

Construction of soft palate defect definitive prosthesis usually starts with a conventional removable prosthesis. Then the palatopharyngeal area is extended to the defect area.[5,18,19] The prosthesis should be designed carefully to accommodate the extra weight and movement of the defect area to provide adequate support, retention, and

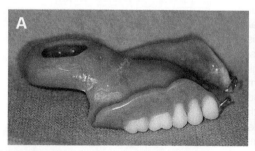
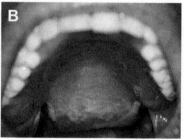

Fig. 6. (*A*) Interim obturator for oropharyngeal defect. The posterior part of the prosthesis was hollowed to decrease its weight. (*B*) Interim obturator for oropharyngeal defect in the patient's mouth.

stability of the prosthesis. The success of the definitive soft palate prosthesis depends on the patient's ability to move the residual muscles of the pharyngeal complex during speech or swallowing. The chance of achieving normal speech is low if the patient exhibits little or no movement of the residual palatopharyngeal complex and they will have hypernasal speech owing to an inability to control nasal emission.[19] In the past for an edentulous patient, the meatus design obturator has historically been recommended.[18,20] The meatus obturator was introduced based on the belief that muscle training in the soft palate area is difficult and may not be success for some patient. Unlike a regular fixed type obturator, this type of obturator ignores the Passavant's pad and the ability of the posterior pharyngeal wall to move. The posterior portion of the meatus obturator extends perpendicular to the hard palate and occludes the airway posterior to the nasal cavity. However, this type of obturator requires extensive clinical experience for their complex clinical procedures.

PROSTHETICS REHABILITATION OF THE ACQUIRED MANDIBULAR DEFECT

Prosthetics rehabilitation of the acquired mandibular defect resulting from oral cancer is very challenging. It requires a good understanding of anatomy and mandibular movement. The extent and location of the mandibular defect, especially the presence or lack of mandibular continuity, are important factors for a favorable outcome.[18,21,22]

Conventional Prosthesis

Continuity defect

Resection of the mandibular body with overlying tissue while maintaining the inferior border of the mandible and its continuity is called marginal mandibulectomy.[22,23] This surgical technique is indicated for head and neck cancer treatment, including cancer of the lower lip, the floor of the mouth, retromolar trigone, gingiva, buccal mucosa, and some skin cancers in the facial area.[23] Soft tissues are used to reconstruct the marginal mandibulectomy such as a skin graft, pedicle graft, or microvascular graft depending on the extension of the resection. Prosthetic rehabilitation after marginal mandibulectomy is less complicated because the continuity of the mandible is maintained and the muscles of mastication are frequently intact.[5,21,22] Conventional removable partial denture type prostheses can enhance a patient's esthetics, improve speech, and provide effective mastication.[21,24]

Owing to the supporting area being compromised, the basic objectives of removable partial denture design is to control and minimize movement of the prosthesis. This minimizes trauma to the reconstructed defect site. The removable partial denture also should have a maximum extension of the denture base and stable occlusion of the prosthesis.[18]

Discontinuity Defects

The prognosis for prosthetic rehabilitation for the patient with a mandibular defect is quite variable. For many patients, reasonable mastication can be achieved, although in some patients only esthetics can be improved.[21] Mandibles lacking continuity are severely compromised biomechanically.[24] All jaw movements and positioning, including resting position, opening, closing, and protruding, are functioning with the remaining muscles around a single load-bearing joint. There are other multiple factors that affect the movement of the discontinuous mandible, for example, the locations of the defect, the number of the remaining teeth, wound healing, and radiation scarring on the defect side.[18,21,25] These factors result in a deviated jaw, a closing movement toward the defect side, and an occlusal discrepancy in the dentate patient.[18,21,25] A specially design removable prosthesis can be fabricated to manage these adverse

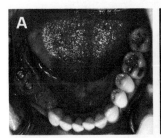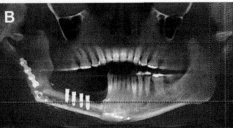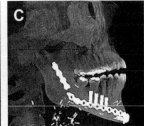

Fig. 7. (*A*) Mandibular defect reconstructed with fibular reconstruction. Intraoral view. Owing to the soft tissue approximation at the surgery, 2 dental implants were used to support the prosthesis. (*B*). Cone beam computed tomography panoramic view. (*C*) Cone beam computed tomography lateral view.

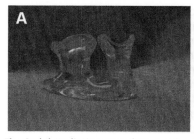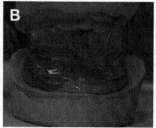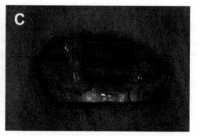

Fig. 8. (*A*) Radiation stent (tongue depression stent). (*B*). Radiation stent in the working cast. (*C*) Radiation stent in the patient's mouth.

outcomes after mandible and tongue surgery and improve function and esthetics for the patient.

COMBINED SURGICAL-PROSTHETIC REHABILITATION

Like the maxillary defect, after cancer resection surgery, an osseocutaneous free flap can be used to reconstruct the mandible.[25] There are multiple available donor sites for free flap reconstruction of the mandible including an osseocutaneous radial forearm free flap, scapula free flap, iliac crest free flap, and the fibula free flap.[26] The fibula free flap provides the greatest bone length, the optimal dimension for a dental implant, and minimal donor site mobility.[26,27] Two surgical teams can work simultaneously at the donor site and recipient site, decreasing the overall operative time. Occasionally, osseointegrated dental implants can also be placed in the same surgery (**Fig. 7**). However, as discussed, the 2-stage approach for dental implant placement is preferred in many institutions. The 2-stage approach minimizes the risk of complications including compromise of the free flap's blood supply. Another advantage of the delayed implant placement approach is to allow the oral and maxillofacial surgeon to place the dental implant in the ideal position and angulation for supporting the mandibular resected prosthesis.

Ancillary Prosthesis for Cancer Therapy

Positioning stents during radiation therapy
Maxillofacial prosthodontists often are asked to fabricate a prosthetic device to support radiation therapy cancer treatment. The design of the device depends on the modality of radiation therapy for the patient with head and neck cancer. In the past, a prosthetic device was necessary to position the radioactive isotopes for brachytherapy.[28] However, as brachytherapy has becoming increasingly rare, the use of these devices has also diminished. External beam radiation with an intensity-modulated radiation therapy technique

has become the treatment of choice for radiation delivery in the head and neck.[28,29] Organ immobilization and the ability to allow repeatable positioning of the patient on daily basis throughout 6 to 8 weeks of radiation therapy are critical for excellent treatment outcome of intensity-modulated radiation therapy (**Fig. 8**).[28,29] Recently, intensity-modulated proton therapy has also been used to treat patients with head and neck cancer.[30] Similar to intensity-modulated radiation therapy, intensity-modulated proton therapy provides a more precise radiation delivery dosage. Positioning stents are often required for this radiation treatment as well. Depending on the location of the tumor and type of radiation therapy, the maxillofacial prosthodontist can design the positioning stent to serve the needs of the radiation oncologist.

Fluoride carrier tray
One of the most common complications during and after radiation therapy for patients with head and neck cancer is salivary gland dysfunction.[31–33] The ionizing radiation causes irreversible damage to the cells of the salivary glands, leaving the

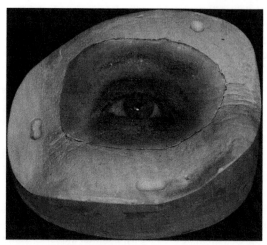

Fig. 9. Orbital prosthesis.

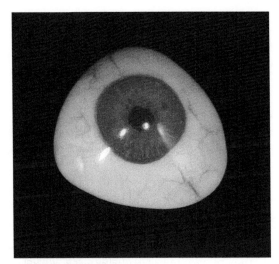

Fig. 10. Ocular prosthesis.

remaining saliva thick and sticky. Patients with salivary gland hypofunction and salivary dysfunction usually have xerostomia, which generally associates with dental caries.[34] This type of dental caries is so-called radiation caries. To prevent radiation caries, a dentate patient who is undergoing and has completed head and neck radiation therapy, topical fluoride treatment is necessary.[31,32,34,35] The patient is counseled to use a high concentration neutral fluoride with a custom mouthpiece application during radiation therapy and to continue this life-long daily topical fluoride treatment after radiation therapy.[31,32,34–37]

Facial Prostheses

As a result of head and neck cancer surgical treatment, some patients require treatment with a facial prosthesis.[38,39] When surgical reconstruction alone cannot fulfill the patient's needs, a facial prosthesis is used to obtain reasonable esthetics of the patient and may also improve function. A facial prosthesis is an artificial replacement of an eye, ear, nose, or other portion of the face that restores normal appearance may improve function (**Figs. 9–12**).[1] The prosthesis is made of medical grade silicone rubber and is custom made to suit the fit and appearance of the individual patient.[33,40] Osseointegrated implants can be placed in strategic maxillofacial areas, which can improve retention and acceptance of facial prostheses.[41]

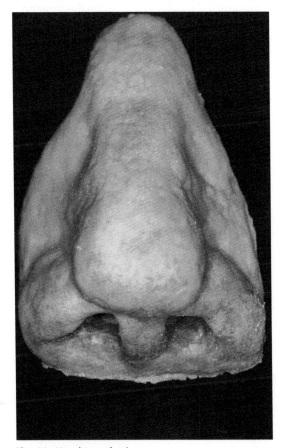

Fig. 11. Nasal prosthesis.

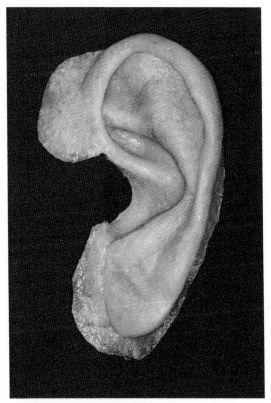

Fig. 12. Auricular prosthesis.

SUMMARY

The treatment of patients with head and neck cancer requires a team approach. Maxillofacial prosthetics are used to support the cancer treatment team during treatment, with oral rehabilitation, and also to improve the patient's quality of life after cancer treatment.

REFERENCES

1. Driscoll CF, Freilich MA, Guckes AD, et al. The glossary of prosthodontic terms. J Prosthet Dent 2017; 117(5):C1-e56.
2. McGuirt WF. Maxillectomy. Otolaryngol Clin North Am 1995;28(6):1175–89.
3. Carrau R. Maxillectomy. Available at: emedicine. medscape.com. Accessed September 23, 2017.
4. Jacob R. Clinical management of the edentulous maxillectomy patient. In: Taylor T, editor. Clinical maxillofacial prosthetics. Chicago: Quintessence Publishing Co, Inc; 2000. p. 85–102.
5. Beumer J III, Marunick M, Garrett N, et al. Rehabilitation of maxillary defects. In: Beumer J III, Marunick M, et al, editors. Maxillofacial rehabilitation: prosthodontic and surgical management of cancer related, acquired, and congenital defects of the head and neck. 3rd edition. Chicago: Quintessence Publishing Co, Inc; 2011. p. 155–210.
6. Arcuri M, Taylor T. Clinical management of the Dentate Maxillectomy Patient. In: Taylor T, editor. Clinical maxillofacial prosthetics. Chicago: Quintessence Publishing Co, Inc; 2000. p. 103–20.
7. Plank D, Weinberg B, Chalian V. Evaluation of speech following prosthetic obturation of surgically acquired maxillary defects. J Prosthet Dent 1981; 45(6):198.
8. Roumanas ED, Nishimura RD, Davis BK, et al. Clinical evaluation of implants retaining edentulous maxillary obturator prostheses. J Prosthet Dent 1997;77(2):184–90.
9. Mericske-Stern R, Perren R, Raveh J. Life table analysis and clinical evaluation of oral implants supporting prostheses after resection of malignant tumors. Int J Oral Maxillofac Implants 1999;14(5):673–80. Available at: http://www.embase.com/search/results?subaction=viewrecord&from=export&id=L129346421%5Cnhttp://sfx.library.uu.nl/utrecht?sid=EMBASE&issn=08822786&id=doi:&atitle=Life+table+analysis+and+clinical+evaluation+of+oral+implants+supporting+prostheses+after+resection.
10. Jaquiéry C, Rohner D, Kunz C, et al. Reconstruction of maxillary and mandibular defects using prefabricated microvascular fibular grafts and osseointegrated dental implants - A prospective study. Clin Oral Implants Res 2004;15(5):598–606.
11. Eckert S, Desjardins R, Taylor T. Clinical management of the soft palate defect. In: Taylor TD, editor. Clinical maxillofacial prosthetics. Quintessence Publishing Co, Inc; 2000. p. 121–31.
12. Drake R, Vogl W, Mitchell A. Gray's anatomy for students. 3rd edition. London (UK): Churchill Livingstone; 2005.
13. Esposito S, Rieger J, Beumer J III. Rehabilitation of soft palate defects. In: Beumer J III, Marunick M, Esposito S, editors. Maxillofacial rehabilitation: prosthodontic and surgical management of cancer related, acquired, and congenital defects of the head and neck. 3rd edition. Chicago: Quintessence Publishing Co, Inc; 2011. p. 213–53.
14. Chambers MS, Lemon JC, Martin JW. Obturation of the partial soft palate defect. J Prosthet Dent 2004; 91(1):75–9.
15. Jones DL. Velopharyngeal function and dysfunction. Clin Commun Disord 1991;1(3):19–25.
16. Witt PD, D'Antonio LL. Velopharyngeal insufficiency and secondary palatal management. A new look at an old problem. Clin Plast Surg 1993;20(4):707–21.
17. Zlotolow I. Restoration of the acquired soft palate deformity with surgical resection and reconstruction. In: Zlotolow I, editor. Proceeding of the first International Congress on Maxillofacial Prosthetics. New York: Memorial Sloan-Kettering Cancer Center; 1995. p. 49–55.
18. Desjardins R, Laney W. Typical clinical problem and approaches to treatment. In: Laney W, editor. Maxillofacial prosthetics. Littleton (CO): PSG Publishing Company; 1979. p. 115–82.
19. Curtis T, Beumer J III. Speech, palatopharyngeal function and restoration of soft palate defects. In: Beumer J III, Curtis T, Firtell D, editors. Maxillofacial rehabilitation: prosthodontic and surgical considerations. St Louis (MO): The C.V. Mosby company; 1979. p. 244–91.
20. Sharry J. Meatus obturator in particular and pharyngeal impression in general. J Prosthet Dent 1958;8: 893–6.
21. Beumer J III, Curtis T. Acquired defects of the mandible. In: Beumer J III, Curtis T, Firtell D, editors. Maxillofacial rehabilitation: prosthodontic and surgical considerations. St. Louis (MO): C V Mosby; 1979. p. 90–187.
22. Taylor T. Diagnostic considerations for prosthodontics rehabilitation of mandibulectomy patient. In: Taylor T, editor. Clinical maxillofacial prosthetics. Chicago (IL): Quintessence Publishing Company; 2000. p. 155–88.
23. Rassekh C. Marginal mandibulectomy. In: Ferris R, editor. Master techniques in otolaryngology-head and neck surgery. Philadelphia: Lippincott Williams and Wilkins; 2013. p. 127–33.
24. Beumer J III, Marunick M, Silverman S Jr. Rehabilitation of tongue and mandibular defects.

In: Beumer J III, Marunick M, Esposito S, editors. Maxillofacial rehabilitation: prosthodontic and surgical management of cancer related, acquired, and congenital defects of the head and neck. 3rd edition. Chicago: Quintessence Publishing Co, Inc; 2011. p. 61–154.

25. Hannam AG, Stavness IK, Lloyd JE, et al. A comparison of simulated jaw dynamics in models of segmental mandibular resection versus resection with alloplastic reconstruction. J Prosthet Dent 2010; 104(3):101–8.

26. Hidalgo DA. Fibula free flap: a new method of mandible reconstruction. Plast Reconstr Surg 1989;84(1):71–9.

27. Pohlenz P, Klatt J, Schön G, et al. Microvascular free flaps in head and neck surgery: complications and outcome of 1000 flaps. Int J Oral Maxillofac Surg 2012;41(6):739–43.

28. Beumer J III. Oral management of patient treated with radiation therapy and/or chemoradiation. In: Beumer J III, Marunick M, Esposito S, editors. Maxillofacial rehabilitation: prosthodontic and surgical management of cancer related, acquired, and congenital defects of the head and neck. 3rd edition. Chicago: Quintessence Publishing Company; 2011. p. 1–60.

29. Lee N, Puri DR, Blanco AI, et al. Intensity-modulated radiation therapy in head and neck cancers: an update. Head Neck 2007;29:387–400.

30. Holliday EB, Frank SJ. Proton radiation therapy for head and neck cancer: a review of the clinical experience to date. Int J Radiat Oncol Biol Phys 2014; 89(2):292–302.

31. Coffin F. The control of radiation caries. Br J Radiol 1973;46(545):365–8.

32. Deech N, Robinson S, Porceddu S, et al. Dental management of patients irradiated for head and neck cancer. Aust Dent J 2014;59(1):20–8.

33. Prosthetics AA of M. Oral health and radiation therapy. Available at: www.maxillofacialprosthetics.org. Accessed September 23, 2017.

34. Jensen SB, Pedersen AML, Vissink A, et al. A systematic review of salivary gland hypofunction and xerostomia induced by cancer therapies: management strategies and economic impact. Support Care Cancer 2010;18(8);1061–70.

35. ADA Division of Communication. Fluoride treatment in dental office. J Am Dent Assoc 2007; 138:420.

36. Englander H. Residual anticaries effect of repeated topical sodium fluoride application by mouth pieces. J Am Dent Assoc 1969;78(4):783–7.

37. Englander HR, Keyes PH, Gestwicki M, et al. Clinical anticaries effect of repeated topical sodium fluoride applications by mouthpieces. J Am Dent Assoc 1967;75(3):638–44.

38. Chalian V. Treating patient with Facial Defect. In: Laney W, editor. Maxillofacial prosthetics. Littleton (CO): PSG Publishing Company; 1979. p. 279–306.

39. Chalian V. Maxillofacial problems involving the use of splint and stents. In: Laney W, editor. Maxillofacial prosthetics. Littleton (CO): PSG Publishing Company; 1979. p. 215–56.

40. Andres C, Haug S. Facial prosthesis fabrication: technical aspect. In: Taylor T, editor. Clinical maxillofacial prosthetics. Chicago (IL): Quintessence Publishing Co, Inc; 2000. p. 233–44.

41. Beumer J III, Reisberg D, Marunick M, et al. Rehabilitation of facial defects. In: Beumer J III, Marunick M, Esposito S, editors. Maxillofacial rehabilitation: prosthodontic and surgical management of cancer related, acquired, and congenital defects of the head and neck. 3rd edition. Chicago: Quintessence Publishing Company; 2011. p. 255–313.

Psychosocial Effects of Head and Neck Cancer

Ali Alias, B.Sc[a,b], Melissa Henry, PhD[c,d],*

KEYWORDS

- Head and neck cancer • Psychosocial • Surgery • Coping • Adaptation • Body image • Function
- Rehabilitation

KEY POINTS

- Head and neck cancer importantly impacts patients' psychological and social well-being.
- The psychosocial effects in the preoperative period cover *coping with symptom discovery and the cancer diagnosis*; *surviving, anticipating functional changes, and information processing*; *communication, patient-physician relationship, and shared decision-making*; and *health behavior change*.
- The postoperative period outlines the following domains: *decisional regret*; *chronic pain*; *posttraumatic stress and fear of cancer recurrence*; *rehabilitation and demoralization*; *disfigurement, dysfunction, and body image concerns*; and *social reintegration*.

This article addresses the perioperative psychosocial aspects of the head and neck cancer (HNC) experience, with implications for clinical practice and future scientific inquiry. The HNC experience can be conceptualized via a *stress-diathesis model*, whereby the stress of being diagnosed with and treated for cancer is understood within and exacerbates the larger context of preexisting biopsychosocial vulnerability.[1] This model is particularly the case in HNC, an illness known for its high levels of anxiety and depression when compared with other oncological populations.[2] Notable stressors faced by patients with HNC include an advanced cancer stage, a high likelihood of cancer recurrence, and extensive treatments involving a high degree of physical symptom burden, disfigurement, and temporary or permanent functional impairments in eating, speech, and breathing. Distress is defined as a "multifactorial unpleasant emotional experience of a psychological (cognitive, behavioral,

emotional), social, and/or spiritual nature that may interfere with the ability to cope with cancer, its physical symptoms and its treatment."[3] In HNC, distress has been shown to compromise a variety of outcomes, including physical rehabilitation and quality of life.

PSYCHOSOCIAL ISSUES IN THE PREOPERATIVE PERIOD

The preoperative period in HNC can be characterized by the following themes: symptom discovery and cancer diagnosis; consenting for treatment; communication and shared decision-making; and health behavior change. The goal of this period is to prepare patients for upcoming treatments and the rehabilitative period.

Symptom Discovery and Cancer Diagnosis

Patients typically experience the HNC diagnosis as life threatening, a sense of alarm that is often

Disclosure Statement: The authors have nothing to disclose.
^a School of Physical and Occupational Therapy, McGill University, Montreal, Quebec, Canada; ^b Faculty of Medicine, McGill University, Montreal, Quebec, Canada; ^c Department of Oncology, Faculty of Medicine, McGill University, Montreal, Quebec, Canada; ^d Department of Oncology and Department of Otolaryngology – Head and Neck Surgery, Jewish General Hospital, 3755 Cote Suite Catherine Road, Pavilion E Room E-872, Montreal, Quebec H3T 1E2, Canada
* Corresponding author. 3755 Cote Suite Catherine Road, Pavilion E Room E-872, Montreal, Quebec H3T 1E2, Canada.
E-mail address: melissa.henry@mcgill.ca

Oral Maxillofacial Surg Clin N Am 30 (2018) 499–512
https://doi.org/10.1016/j.coms.2018.06.010
1042-3699/18/© 2018 Elsevier Inc. All rights reserved.

further exacerbated by an advanced stage and life-altering treatments. Diagnostic delays may be experienced with regret and/or anger, as signs may have been minimized until symptoms evolved and/or interfered with the patients' functioning, secondary to the patients' help-seeking habits, low health literacy, misinterpretation of symptoms (eg, tooth ache/dental pain, allergies, or common cold), avoidance-based coping, refusal of having their life interrupted, other life stressors, and/or system delays in referrals.[4]

Patients often experience a variety of emotions, such as fear of mortality, uncertainty about the future, and social concerns.[5] The ambiguity can persist after the diagnosis, as future tests may be needed to determine the extent of the disease, with corollary readjustments made to the treatment plan. The visible impact of treatments on body structures and functioning are not always foreseeable, adding to the uncertainty and requiring flexibility to readjust to unanticipated events.[6] Lazarus's[7] "Transactional Model of Stress and Coping" defines coping behavior as "constantly changing cognitive and behavioral efforts to manage specific demands that are appraised as taxing or exceeding the resources of the person."[7] Coping skills become important as patients assimilate diagnostic- and treatment-related information and are faced with often unwanted changes in appearance and vital functions, considered a trade-off for survival.[8]

Appreciating the cause of HNC is of interest as it relates to coping. HNCs showcase 2 streams: squamous cell carcinoma (SCC), related to tobacco and alcohol use, and human papillomavirus (HPV). An increased clinical incidence of HPV-positive oropharyngeal carcinomas has been noted, requiring an appreciation of the particularities in the experience of SCC- and HPV-related HNCs.[9–11] HPV-positive oropharyngeal patients tend to be younger, with less exposure to alcohol and tobacco, higher socioeconomic status, and higher responsiveness to treatments.[12] Although the prognosis of HPV-positive HNCs is much better than HPV-negative HNCs, their interpersonal nature requires attention.[13] As HPV is often sexually transmitted, patients often need guidance to understand how they contracted HPV, especially as the diagnosis can lead them to reexamine past life behaviors and question couple fidelity. Patients may need information on partner risk, help to address issues around social stigma, and work out potential stress in the patient-caregiver dyad.[6,14] On the other side of the spectrum of cause, patients with alcohol- and/or tobacco-related SCC HNC can exhibit personality traits, such as neuroticism/lack of flexibility,

dependency, and lower adaptive coping by over-reliance on denial, avoidance, and substance use.[14,15] Although denial can be a normal initial response to the diagnosis of cancer, its persistent use accompanied by avoidance can interfere with decision-making and self-care, in turn impeding medical outcomes. As part of routine management, patients exhibiting early signs of enduring denial and avoidance should be properly evaluated and followed using a collaborative care model, including consultation liaison and psychosocial oncology services.[2] Clinicians should also be attentive to cognitive impairments and involve geriatric medicine as needed to minimize delays and optimize the medical and psychosocial management of the disease.[16,17]

The role of anxiety preoperatively can be explained by cognitive models of anxiety, which propose that attentional biases in the processing of life-threatening information are a primary factor in the cause and maintenance of acute anxiety.[18] These attentional biases consist of a difficulty to disengage attention from the threatening stimuli, impacting the potential to engage in coping.[18] Continuous stressors will further exacerbate the response. The panoply of information concerning disease cause, prognosis, medical management (eg, secondary/reconstructive surgeries, concomitant radiotherapy/chemotherapy), and ensuing complications/side effects in body impairments, activity limitations, and participation restrictions plays an important role in the psychological response. Common reactions include fear, worry, and anguish, which may intersect with feelings of vulnerability, heightening the anxious response and in some cases resulting in a sense of hopelessness and demoralization, as patients may feel at an impasse.[8] Although a cancer diagnosis is undeniably stressful for all, patients with high levels of anxiety or other known markers for vulnerability should routinely be provided with the opportunity for psychological support from the moment of diagnosis to help build resources for coping.

Consenting for Treatment in the Context of a Life-Threatening Disease

The preoperative period requires patients to assimilate information and make complex decisions.[19,20] The capacity for informed consent, defined as a treatment-related decision taking into account the current status and postoperative consequences, may be diminished because of the patients' intrinsic desire to survive taking precedence and potentially reinforcing an attentional bias.[21] As human information processing capacity is limited, selective attention allows one to avoid information overload by prioritizing certain information, leading to temporal discounting (ie, the tendency to discount future consequences and focus on immediate demands).[22] Some patients may rush toward curative treatment without full consideration of its effects, negatively impacting the postoperative rehabilitation period as patients feel ill prepared.

Additionally, the acute stress and associated insomnia risks affecting executive functioning, involving the capacity to reason, problem solve, and anticipate,[23] in turn negatively impacting emotional regulation and the flexibility required to adapt to stressful situations, potentially compromising patients' decision-making participation. The cause of neurocognitive repercussions in oncology is multifactorial and has yet to be fully elaborated; however, certain mechanisms have been proposed, including the stress-induced responses as seen through the *framework on stress reactivity*.[24] This framework posits that the brain maintains allostasis (ie, homeostasis through adaption to stressors); its overuse leads to dysregulation, coined allostatic load, and underlying neurophysiologic changes in response to chronic stress. These changes limit the ability to use cognitive resources for the purpose of adaptation and coping due to the dysregulated states of biochemical (eg, cortisol), neurophysiologic (eg, hypothalamic-pituitary-adrenal axis), and functional systems (eg, prefrontal cortex). Other mechanisms may include genetic polymorphisms, whereby a subgroup of patients present with a genetic predisposition toward stress reactivity.[24] Providing patients with early support may help regulate an overactive neurophysiologic stress response and, in turn, not only help alleviate unbearable stress but also help expand the cognitive resources necessary for informed consent.[25] Early support is in recognizing that patients may value differently their preoperative decision in the postsurgical period, when they are faced with their altered body. Slowing down the process, while respecting the need for a timely decision and treatment plan, can help prepare patients for what lies ahead and attenuate its trauma.

When inadequately tailored, the extent and format of information presented to patients can also compound stress-induced responses, restricting any preexisting capacity to anticipate what it would be like to experience the suggested, often abstract, impairments. Physicians ought to be attuned to their patients' emotional state, include family caregivers in the consultation room when appropriate to increase information recall and assimilation, and use good communication skills to help patients in decision-making.[19,26,27]

Communication and Shared Decision-Making

Communication is an essential component of care, requiring an understanding of patients as dynamic entities whose values and decisions may fluctuate throughout the HNC trajectory.[19] The higher ratio of male patients often seen in HNC means that distress may be less readily identifiable, which is of concern, as rates of psychological distress and suicidal ideations are high in HNC.[2] The literature on masculinity and decision-making refers to the underlying value of autonomy, which may not be responsive to an authoritarian clinical approach.[28] Men may also display a particular way of processing information with an orientation toward problem-solving, self-reliance, and action, a tendency that can be reinforced in a busy head and neck oncology clinic, as time is limited and the care can be fragmented into a step-by-step approach limiting a more longitudinal viewpoint. As each patient is different, an understanding of the patients' personal traits and preferences should be appreciated to tailor patient-clinician interactions accordingly. This understanding requires clinicians to stay mindful of the patients' reality and of the patients' way of coping and emotional regulation and to readjust their pace of communication accordingly.

There is strong evidence encouraging clinicians to be explicit in their presentation of medical information. A common model for physician communication is the *Ask-Tell-Ask Framework* (**Table 1**).[19] The first *ask* consists of asking patients an open-ended question about their understanding and what they would like to know (eg, What do you understand of your cancer? What do you understand of your surgery?). The patients *tell*, providing the physician knowledge on their level of understanding and on their concerns. The last *ask* consists of permission to talk about an important topic and to clarify the patients' understanding considering the new information. This method allows one to address misconceptions and engages patients in the decision-making process by encouraging their sense of control and authority.[19]

During the provision of life-threatening information, patients process via 2 channels: an emotional and a cognitive channel.[19] The delivery of this information should be without interruption and needs to show empathy, as emotional reactions may occur instantaneously. Clinicians should refrain from filling silences with further information, as the emotional channel overrides the cognitive channel, impacting the patients' capacity to understand the presented information.[19] Communication can be further facilitated with the use of decision aids in the form of pamphlets, videos,

Table 1	
The ask-tell-ask framework	
Concept	Description
Ask	• The health care provider seeks to understand the patients' baseline knowledge about their proposed treatment and what they would like to know.
	• The health care provider formulates open-ended questions.
	• Example: What do you understand of your cancer? What would you like to know about your treatment/impacts on appearance and function/rehabilitation?
Tell	• The patients describe what they understand and the information they would like to know.
	• This step seeks to engage patients in the decision-making process, by helping patients consider the pros and cons of the presented treatment options.
Ask	• The health care provider asks for permission to clarify the patients' understanding and to provide additional information relative to the impacts of the proposed treatments.
	• This step seeks to encourage the patients' sense of autonomy.

The Ask-Tell-Ask Framework. The Ask-Tell-Ask framework is also available at http://vitaltalk.org/topics/establish-rapport/?vtitle=ask-tell-ask.

Data from Beers E, Nilsen ML, Johnson JT. The role of patients: shared decision-making. Otolaryngol Clin North Am 2017;50(4):689–708.

and Web-based platforms. These tools can be an effective means of increasing patient knowledge and risk perception and reducing decisional conflict and passivity in decision-making.[29]

These evidence-based frameworks ensure a common ground between patients and clinicians, paving the way for shared decision-making.[19] Shared treatment-related decision-making denotes 4 steps: informing patients, explaining treatment options, identifying patients' values/goals, and making a mutual decision. Each step has a particular importance; a breach in a single step (eg, misinformation arising from Internet consultation, unclear presentation of prognosis) can cause a misaligned decision, potentially impacting the patient-physician alliance.[19] There is a paucity of literature discussing optimal ways to address patient preferences and allow patient participation within the HNC decision-making context.[26] Patients with HNC are usually faced with a limited

number of treatment options that they either accept or refuse, casting the physician in an authoritarian rather than collaborative role. Minimally, to render this process patient centered, one needs to appreciate the characteristics of individuals (eg, sex, culture, medical literacy) and their milieu (eg, social support) to tailor the communicative approach and allow patient participation even in the face of limited options.[19,26]

Generally, patients can be allocated to 3 categories of decision-making: active, collaborative, or passive.[30] Active patients make the final decision following clinical recommendations; collaborative patients ensure equal responsibility within the patient-physician framework; and passive patients require the physician to play a central decision-making role. Active patients are generally seen to be younger, more educated, of higher socioeconomic status, and require more information as they search for full participation in decision-making. An authoritarian approach risks threatening these patients' autonomy. Patients who are older, non-Caucasian, and of lower socioeconomic status generally tend to be more passive decision makers and showcase important knowledge gaps, as they tend to rely on the treating team. These gaps suggest that patients may not be wary of postoperative repercussions and, hence, may be prone to experience decisional regrets. Thus, the HNC team needs to balance an approach to patients that will include free and informed consent as well as be based on their values and preferences, verifying patients' understanding of the cancer, the treatment options, and associated repercussions on appearance and function. A misalignment of decision-making styles may ultimately compromise satisfaction with care and undermine confidence in the treating team, having far-reaching consequences, such as impacting the patients' compliance with treatments, interfering with future medical decisions, and augmenting the risk of litigation.[19,31]

Health Behavior Change

As tobacco and alcohol account for an estimated 75% of HNC diagnoses, the HNC care trajectory is accompanied by recommendations for substance use abstinence in the service of reducing recurrences, symptom burden, treatment complications, and mortality.[32] The process of modifying one's behavior can be seen through the *transtheoretical model of health behavior change*, involving 6 stages of change: precontemplation, contemplation, preparation, action, maintenance, and termination (**Table 2**).[33] Individuals progress through these stages, which are influenced by

Table 2	
The constructs of the transtheoretical model of health behavior change	
Stages of Change	**Description**
Precontemplation	No intention to take action within the next 6 mo
Contemplation	Intends to take action within the next 6 mo
Preparation	Intends to take action within the next 30 d and has taken some behavioral steps in this direction
Action	Changed overt behavior for <6 mo
Maintenance	Changed overt behavior for more than 6 mo
Termination	No temptation to relapse and 100% confidence

From Prochaska J, Redding C, Evers K. The transtheoretical model and stages of change. In: Glanz K, Rimer BK, Viswanath K, editors. Health behavior and health education: theory, research, and practice. 4th edition. San Francisco (CA): Jossey-Bass; 2008. p. 98–9; with permission.

Box 1

The FRAMES approach for treatment of substance use

- *Feedback* is given to the individual about personal risk or impairment.
- *Responsibility* for change is placed on the participant.
- *Advice* to change is given by the provider.
- *Menu* of alternative self-help or treatment options is offered to the participant.
- *Empathetic* style is used in counseling.
- *Self-efficacy* or optimistic empowerment is engendered in the participant

From Center for Substance Abuse Treatment. Brief interventions and brief therapies for substance abuse, treatment improvement protocol series, no. 34. Rockville (VA): Substance Abuse and Mental Health Services Administration; 1999. p. 16.

---

decisional balance (the weighing of pros and cons of changing), *self-efficacy* (situation-specific confidence when coping without relapsing to the unhealthy habit), and *temptations* (the intensity of the urges to engage in a habit).[33]

As patients may present with an important pack-year and alcohol consumption history, behavior change can be demanding because of habituation and low levels of self-efficacy and adaptive coping, especially preoperatively when these substances may be used for stress relief. Despite the large proportion of patients with HNC who attempt to quit before treatment, a substantial amount relapse, highlighting barriers to cessation maintenance.[34] Barriers to address in follow-ups include the immediate effects of cessation, risk perception, withdrawal symptoms, physical symptom burden, psychological distress, lack of information on the impacts beyond cancer recurrence, and an authoritarian approach in counseling.[34,35] As continued substance use has been associated with compromised medical outcomes, an important focus should be given to substance cessation, with an emphasis on posttreatment follow-up to reinforce maintenance. Clinical practice guidelines need to be systematically applied, including the use of brief interventions, such as the 5 A's and FRAMES (feedback, responsibility, advice, menu, empathy, and self-efficacy) approaches (**Box 1**, **Fig. 1**,

respectively). These brief interventions aim to investigate a problem in a short patient-clinician interaction, whereby motivational strategies are used in a step-by-step fashion to reinforce the patients' motivation to change their health behavior and whereby the patients are connected with evidence-based resources to increase the chances of success and reduce the likelihood of negative consequences (eg, withdrawal, relapse). Motivational interviewing, medical aids (eg, nicotine replacement therapy, medication facilitating alcohol abstinence), and behavioral counseling (eg, 12-Steps approach, alcohol rehabilitation center, couple/family therapy) are other therapeutic options.[36] The combination of behavioral counseling with medical aids and routine follow-ups is ideal for promoting long-term cessation.[37]

As patients abstain from tobacco and alcohol, either voluntarily or because of a functional impairment, one needs to be wary of chemical coping, defined as the use of opioids (and/or other psychotropic medications) to cope with life stressors.[38] The use of narcotic analgesics for coping purposes is of concern, as outlined by recent literature suggesting a link between opioid prescription in cancer pain management and anxiety, major depressive disorder, and substance use disorder.[39] One may also want to consider genetic susceptibility to addiction, as patients presenting with certain genotypes may warrant a specific approach to pain management.[40] Ultimately, an assessment of patients' medication and substance use history, as well as their psychosocial well-being, allows proper

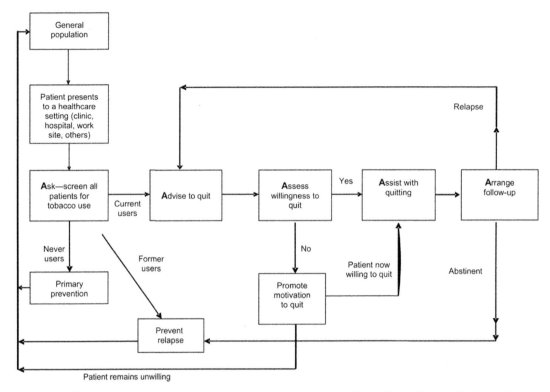

Fig. 1. The 5 A's model for treatment of tobacco use and dependence. (*From* Clinical Practice Guideline Treating Tobacco Use and Dependence 2008 Update Panel, Liaisons, and Staff. A clinical practice guideline for treating tobacco use and dependence: 2008 update: a U.S. public health service report. Am J Prev Med 2008;35(2):162; with permission.)

targeting of the suffering and sets the stage for optimal treatment outcomes. Apart from alcohol and nicotine abstinence, patients can be encouraged to become physically active; maintain a healthy diet, weight, and good dental hygiene; and ensure ultraviolet protection.[8] In addition to encouraging physical fitness and function, these initiatives can help patients maintain a sense of control and order in the face of adversity. These motivators are non-negligible motivators that are proximal to patients' concerns as functioning in their daily activities and roles is central to them.[34]

PSYCHOSOCIAL ISSUES IN THE POSTOPERATIVE PERIOD

Following the acute cancer treatment phase, patients enter a rehabilitation period whereby their focus shifts toward recovering function.[34,41] The impact of functional losses can be seen through the World Health Organization's *International Classification of Functioning, Disability, and Health* (ICF), which provides a comprehensive perspective of the implications for body impairments, activity limitations, and participation restrictions

(**Fig. 2**). This framework defines function as more than its strictly physical understanding and takes into account medical, personal, and environmental factors that play a mediating role in limiting and/or facilitating the experience of impairments, limitations, and restrictions.

Rehabilitation can be seen through the 5-dimensional framework of the *Rehab-CYCLE*.[42] Starting with the *identification of the problems and needs*, this cycle proceeds to *relate the problems to modifiable and limiting factors*; to *define target problems, mediators, and select appropriate measures*; to *plan the interventions*; to *assess the effects*; and, lastly, to *reidentify other problems and needs*. This framework along with the ICF provides a patient-centered perspective on impaired functioning, outlining areas (body structures/functions, activities, participations) that require rehabilitation.[43] Clinicians need to be wary of the difficult survivorship period; the transition from illness to health, however noteworthy, may become difficult because of symptom clusters including pain, fatigue, anxiety, and depression.[32] Postoperatively, psycho-oncology services may assist patients to attain the best outcomes by providing the necessary support to improve function and help adjust

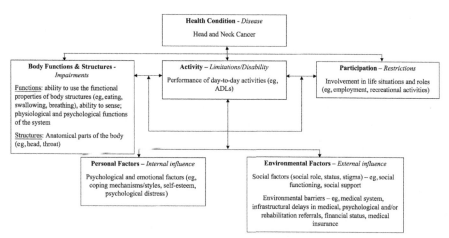

Fig. 2. World Health Organization's ICF using an example in head and neck oncology. ADLs, activities of daily living. (*Adapted from* World Health Organization (WHO). Towards a common language for functioning, disability and health: ICF (The International Classification of Functioning, Disability and Health). p. 9. Available at: http://www.who.int/classifications/icf/training/icfbeginnersguide.pdf. Accessed January 20, 2018; with permission.)

expectations, allowing patients to flexibly adjust to their state of limitations.[44] In the postoperative period, main psychosocial themes include *decisional regrets*; *pain management*; *posttraumatic stress and the fear of cancer recurrence*; *rehabilitation, depression, and demoralization*; and *disfigurement, dysfunction, body image concerns, and social reintegration*.

Decisional Regrets

As patients cope with the HNC aftermath, they may exhibit decisional regrets as they navigate through rehabilitation.[45] Risk factors associated with decisional regret include higher pretreatment decisional conflict, lower treatment-related satisfaction, adverse functioning, and greater anxiety levels.[46] Regrets involving life habits (eg, substance use) can resurface and take the form of self-blame, which apart from affecting well-being can bring patients to delay symptom reporting because of feelings of shame and guilt. Decisional regrets arising from functional and cosmetic outcomes may impact the patient-physician relationship, especially when there is a discrepancy between initial expectations and actual medical outcomes[45] or when there is misalignment between patients' perception of the outcome and their physician's intentionally supportive, but perceived as overly positive (and potentially minimizing), discourse.

The *Cognitive-Social Health Information-Processing model* can be useful to further understand decisional regrets.[47,48] This model seeks to analyze how individuals cognitively and affectively process information about their health, medical risks, and treatment options and how this information translates into health-enhancing or health-defeating behavior. It indicates that the individual's health-related values and self-regulatory capacities (eg, capacity for self-management and emotional regulation) interact dynamically with distress to produce specific patterns of responses in light of health challenges. Thus, patients who are high on self-monitoring (ie, attend and amplify symptom clusters, functional and cosmetic outcomes) are likely to exhibit higher levels of distress, in turn heightening decisional regrets after treatment, as rehabilitation is lengthy and the extent of recovery is ambiguous. To reduce decisional regret, one would need to work on improving patients' self-regulatory capacities, all the while ensuring proper physical rehabilitation and symptom management.[45] One needs to provide patients with early support when experiencing decisional regret in order to maximize function.

Pain Management

A meta-analysis identified pain in 57% (95% confidence interval [CI] = 43%–70%) of patients with HNC before treatment and in 42% (95% CI = 33%–50%) after treatment.[49] Pain in HNC includes inflammatory, nociceptive, and neuropathic components.[50] HNC pain has been generally associated with younger age, female sex, lower income, advanced stage, surgery, and radiotherapy.[49] Although pain is a direct function of the tumor's and treatment's effect, it has been found to intensify as a result of psychosocial (eg, psychological distress, cultural and pain beliefs, coping responses), behavioral (eg, substance use), and biological factors (eg, sensory input).[51]

Chronic pain is a distressing and disabling symptom present in up to 40% of patients with HNC, impacting their social reintegration.[52] It is often accompanied by difficulties in coping, as manifested by pain catastrophizing, and fear of injury.[51] Chronic pain may be heightened by (and reciprocally potentiate) psychological distress, as both have an interplay in neurophysiologic feedback loops, implying the need to apprehend the multidimensional construct of *total pain*.[32] This construct emphasizes the screening of pain through a symptom cluster perspective, including assessments of fatigue, anxiety, depression, and sleep disturbances.[32] A routine assessment of pain will ensure the provision of multimodal approaches (eg, pharmacologic, psychological, social, and integrative) conducive to addressing the root sources of the suffering. Patient education on the prevalence and management of pain should be considered, especially in the context of stigmatized attitudes toward opioids (eg, stigma, fear of addiction or of opioid overdose) and psychiatric medications.[50] Refusal to take opioids and/or psychiatric medication can become problematic when patients are noncompliant to medical recommendations that would otherwise improve prognosis and facilitate functional recovery. In these cases, motivational interviewing combined with psychoeducation can help patients move from *contemplation* to *planning* in the cycle of adopting a new behavior, such as the use of analgesics and/or psychiatric medication.[33] Pharmacologic management of pain should consider frameworks such as the World Health Organization's *Analgesic Ladder* to stratify pain with the appropriate level of

intervention, varying from nonsteroidal antiinflammatory drugs to opioid medication, and including adjuvants, such as antiepileptic drugs, antianxiety and antidepressant medication (**Fig. 3**).[53] Behavioral approaches that have also shown to be effective in pain management include coping skills training, hypnosis, and cognitive-behavioral therapy (eg, reframing catastrophizing thoughts, relaxation with guided imagery).[54] Structured physical exercise during anticancer treatment can also be considered in optimizing medical outcomes and in shifting the patients' thoughts and emotional responses.[55,56]

Posttraumatic Stress and the Fear of Cancer Recurrence

Following surgery, patients may require radiotherapy. Common radiotherapy-related stressors include claustrophobia due to immobilization with a mask and the confined and isolated space.[57] Patients with a history of trauma may especially experience stress in these circumstances, with the re-experiencing of trauma and emerging issues around trust and isolation. Fear of recurrence is another cancer-specific form of anxiety in which reminders of the traumatic experience may potentiate anxiety-induced responses. Although its prevalence is not well documented, a longitudinal HNC study found that 35% of patients presented this fear during the cancer trajectory.[58] HNC may enhance fear of cancer recurrence considering its prognosis, posttreatment symptoms similar to those of the cancer discovery, and close monitoring through follow-up visits and medical imaging.

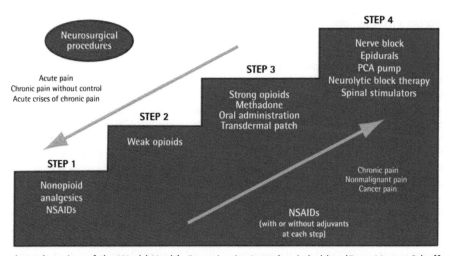

Fig. 3. An adapted version of the World Health Organization's analgesic ladder. (*From* Vargas-Schaffer G. Is the WHO analgesic ladder still valid? Can Fam Physician 2010;56(6):516; with permission; and *Adapted from* World Health Organization. Cancer pain ladder for adults. Available at: http://www.who.int/cancer/palliative/painladder/en/. Accessed January 4, 2018; with permission.)

The cancer experience has been found sufficiently traumatic to induce posttraumatic stress disorder symptoms among a minority of cancer survivors, especially in HNC, whereby the disease and treatments are a stressful assault on the body and patients are confronted with constant social reminders.[5] Posttraumatic stress disorder develops in the context of a traumatic event that threatens one's well-being, causing individuals to react with helplessness or shock and after which they reexperience memories and emotions through sensory flashbacks and nightmares.[5] Individuals are seen to avoid reminders of the trauma and become emotionally numb, anxious, and hypervigilant. These symptoms are described as clinical when they cause significant suffering and impact functioning. Current prevalence of cancer-related posttraumatic stress disorder is noted to be of 6.4% (95% CI = 4.1%–9.9%), lifetime of 12.6% (95% CI = 7.4%–20.7%), and subsyndromal of 10% to 20%.[59] Evidence shows that posttraumatic stress disorder in patients with cancer increases morbidity and mortality, notably playing a key role in the experience and response to pain. Risk factors among cancer survivors include lifetime history of psychiatric disorders and trauma, low socioeconomic status, young age, limited social support, advanced disease, invasive treatment, and a heightened threat perception.[5,59] In conjunction with antianxiety medication, evidence-based management of posttraumatic stress disorder includes trauma-based cognitive-behavioral therapy (ie, exposure-based treatments, such as systematic desensitization, applied relaxation, and cognitive therapy whereby patients are probed to explore and alter the threat appraisals that maintain the phobic valence) and eye movement desensitization and reprocessing (ie, a technique using eye movement and other bilateral stimulation to help in the reprocessing of traumatic events).[60]

Furthermore, the caregiver's well-being, the concept of dyadic coping, and their effects on the patients' rehabilitation should not be overlooked.[6] Caregivers are known to experience significant emotional distress, with recurrence fears and posttraumatic stress arising from being traumatized in their exposure to the pain and suffering of patients and their caregiving roles involving pain management, dressing changes, food preparation, and enteral feeding.[5] During the treatment phase, patients often become dependent on their caregivers for daily activities. As they physically improve, some patients may resist reclaiming autonomy, independence, and role resumption, with underlying feelings of insecurity and vulnerability arising from the traumatic cancer experience.[8] Some caregivers may also have trouble letting go of their role. Furthermore, the interplay of treatment effects and stigma may limit patients and partners approaching topics of intimacy and sexuality with the treating team.[61] Patients may feel the need to protect themselves from physical contact because of the development of a new sense of body vulnerability.

Rehabilitation, Depression, and Demoralization

Physical rehabilitation from HNC treatments is often a slow-paced process, with patients experiencing a sense of uncertainty, as functional recovery is usually thought to be longer than expected.[8] This sense of stagnation may act as a catalyst for the development of demoralization, in part explaining why depression peaks in patients with HNC postoperatively.[62,63] In fact, the prevalence of major depressive disorder in HNC is 9.2%, whereas adjustment disorder with depressed mood is reported at 16.3%.[64] Clinicians need to be attentive to signs of demoralization and refer to psychosocial oncology services accordingly. These signs include lowered morale, perceived incapacity to cope, hopelessness, and a loss of meaning and self-worth. The experience of demoralization has been associated with the wish to hasten death and suicidal thoughts, which can be directly or indirectly communicated.[65]

Other explanations proposed to account for posttreatment depressive symptoms in HNC include morbidities associated with advanced staging (eg, functional/performance status, cognitive decline); dysregulation of the hypothalamic-pituitary-adrenal axis[24]; hypothyroidism after radiotherapy[66]; a life history of depressive disorder[67]; a personality with high levels of neuroticism precluding flexibility to readjust to the multiple transitions involved in HNC[67]; a transdiagnostic hypothesis whereby anxiety on diagnosis and depression after treatment share common genetic, familial, and environmental susceptibility[68,69]; and the existential angst and awareness that comes with treatment-related physical symptoms.[70] No matter the cause, depression and demoralization need to be identified and properly treated by specialists in psychosocial oncology to improve medical outcomes, including survival.[71]

Disfigurement, Dysfunction, Body Image Concerns, and Social Reintegration

Despite advances in surgical techniques, patients' appearance can still be altered following HNC surgery.[70] The impact of disfigurement and functional impairments can have important repercussions on the patients' self-esteem, body image, interpersonal relationships, and communication. Patients may experience social anxiety, accompanied by intrusive thoughts, hypervigilance, and/or avoidant behaviors,[72] which may be exacerbated by stigmatized public reactions.[73]

Of concern is the construct of body image, which is defined as a subjective and dynamic concept, including one's perceptions, feelings, and behaviors toward the body and function.[74,75] Body image concerns in oncology can be seen through a framework integrating the ICF with oncology-specific concepts of body image disturbances (ie, self-perception of a change in appearance and/or function and lack of satisfaction with the alteration and psychological distress regarding changes in appearance and/or function).[76] This framework represents the multidimensional nature of body image concerns in oncology whereby impairments in body functions/structures, activity limitations, and participation restrictions may impact one's sense of self.[77] Body image concerns can also be viewed as a manifestation of postoperative depression due to its associated negative self-perception. According to White's *heuristic model of body image dimensions*, following a perceived change, patients remodel their body schema to integrate their current physical and functional state with their body ideals, which often need to be reshaped according to their new reality (**Fig. 4**).[78] This process of recovery can require much effort, especially when an important value was ascribed to the altered and/or lost feature/function. An ideal-self discrepancy may be present and demonstrated by automatic thoughts (eg, self-discrimination, self-stigma),

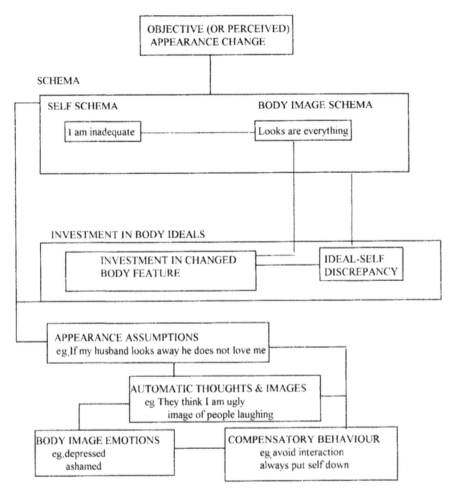

Fig. 4. A heuristic model of body image dimensions following an objective or perceived change in appearance. (*From* White CA. Body image dimensions and cancer: a heuristic cognitive behavioral model. Psychooncology 2000;9(3):187; with permission.)

emotions (eg, shock, shame, sadness), and compensatory behaviors (eg, avoiding interaction and/or intimacy). This sense of vulnerability will have a toll on the patients' rehabilitation, as this discrepancy will require them to reinvest and reintegrate their body ideals to align with their current status. Indicators of body image concerns include unrealistic expectations about outcomes, decision-making difficulties due to appearance concerns, persistent dissatisfaction and avoidance of viewing oneself postoperatively, and avoidance of social situations.[75]

Throughout the process of recovery, patients may *mourn the loss*, *confront the loss*, *confront possible denial*, *reframe the experience*, and *integrate the experience*.[79] This perspective on recovery is patient specific, as each process may be experienced several times during the survivorship period. Furthermore, *the 3 C's framework* can be used to approach body image topics with patients.[75] Postoperatively, clinicians should especially take the time to normalize patients' concerns by reminding them that body image disturbances are *common* after cancer and usually resolve with time. Clinicians should then invite patients to explore their body image *concerns* as well as ask patients about the *consequences* of these concerns on their daily functioning. To address body image disturbances, evidence supports referral to appropriate specialists for psychosocial support using, for example, cognitive-behavioral therapy, including psychoeducation, cognitive restructuring, desensitization, and social skills training.[74,75]

SUMMARY

This article underlines the importance of perioperative psychological issues in the HNC trajectory continuum. It underlines the importance of screening for distress and of an integrated collaborative approach to optimize medical and quality-of-life outcomes in this population. Routine distress screening is required at specific time points in the HNC trajectory (eg, first occurrence, recurrence or progression of HNC, after surgery, during radiation and after radiation therapy, and at regular intervals during the follow-up period).[2,80] A stepped-care model can be used to ensure best practices are in place for the management of psychosocial concerns, particularly in areas of anxiety, depression, and suicide risk.[69,81,82] There are different trajectories of psychological responses, ranging from those affected by disease and treatment (ie, stress) to those that enter treatment with vulnerability (ie, diathesis, genetic sensitivity), and others presenting with both (ie, diathesis-stress).[1]

Further research should focus on mechanisms underlying distress to better delineate tailored and personalized intervention modalities. Addressing psychological distress is important to optimize outcomes in this vulnerable population.

REFERENCES

1. Ronde R, Plomin R. Diathesis-stress models of psychopathology: a quantitative genetic perspective. Appl Prev Psychol 1992;1(4):177–82.
2. Williams Charlene C. Psychosocial distress and distress screening in multidisciplinary head and neck cancer treatment. Otolaryngol Clin North Am 2017;50(4):807–23.
3. National Comprehensive Cancer Network. Distress management. Clinical practice guidelines. J Natl Compr Canc Netw 2003;1(3):344–74.
4. Goy J, Hall SF, Feldman-Stewart D, et al. Diagnostic delay and disease stage in head and neck cancer: a systematic review. Laryngoscope 2009;119(5):889–98.
5. Cordova MJ, Riba MB, Spiegel D. Post-traumatic stress disorder and cancer. Lancet Psychiatry 2017;4(4):330–8.
6. Sterba KR, Zapka J, Armeson KE, et al. Physical and emotional well-being and support in newly diagnosed head and neck cancer patient-caregiver dyads. J Psychosoc Oncol 2017;35(6):646–65.
7. Lazarus RS. The psychology of stress and coping. Issues Ment Health Nurs 1985;7(1–4):399–418.
8. Cohen EE, LaMonte SJ, Erb NL, et al. American Cancer Society Head and Neck Cancer survivorship care guideline. CA Cancer J Clin 2016;66(3):203–39.
9. Chaturvedi AK, Engels EA, Pfeiffer RM, et al. Human papillomavirus and rising oropharyngeal cancer incidence in the United States. J Clin Oncol 2011;29(32):4294–301.
10. Reich M, Licitra L, Vermorken JB, et al. Best practice guidelines in the psychosocial management of HPV-related head and neck cancer: recommendations from the European Head and Neck Cancer Society's make sense campaign. Ann Oncol 2016;27(10):1848–54.
11. Dodd RH, Waller J, Marlow LA. Human papillomavirus and head and neck cancer: psychosocial impact in patients and knowledge of the link - a systematic review. Clin Oncol (R Coll Radiol) 2016;28(7):421–39.
12. Chu KP, Habbous S, Kuang Q, et al. Socioeconomic status, human papillomavirus, and overall survival in head and neck squamous cell carcinomas in Toronto, Canada. Cancer Epidemiol 2016;40:102–12.
13. Ang KK, Harris J, Wheeler R, et al. Human papillomavirus and survival of patients with oropharyngeal cancer. N Engl J Med 2010;363(1):24–35.

14. Giuliani M, Milne R, McQuestion M, et al. Partner's survivorship care needs: an analysis in head and neck cancer patients. Oral Oncol 2017;71:113–21.

15. Morris N, Moghaddam N, Tickle A, et al. The relationship between coping style and psychological distress in people with head and neck cancer: a systematic review. Psychooncology 2018;27(3): 734–47.

16. Williams AM, Lindholm J, Siddiqui F, et al. Clinical assessment of cognitive function in patients with head and neck cancer: prevalence and correlates. Otolaryngol Head Neck Surg 2017;157(5):808–15.

17. Kunkel EJ, Woods CM, Rodgers C, et al. Consultations for 'maladaptive denial of illness' in patients with cancer: psychiatric disorders that result in noncompliance. Psychooncology 1997;6(2):139–49.

18. Stöber J. Anxiety: the cognitive perspective, by Michael W. Eysenck Hove, UK: Lawrence erlbaum; 1992; 195 pp. Anxiety, Stress, Coping 1993;6(2): 149–50.

19. Beers E, Lee Nilsen M, Johnson JT. The role of patients: shared decision-making. Otolaryngol Clin North Am 2017;50(4):689–708.

20. Main BG, McNair AGK, Haworth S, et al. Core information set for informed consent to surgery for oral or oropharyngeal cancer: a mixed-methods study. Clin Otolaryngol 2018;43(2):624–31.

21. Sharpe L, Thewes B, Butow P. Attentional biases in cancer survivors: directions for future research. Psychooncology 2015;24(4):496.

22. Franco-Watkins AM, Mattson RE, Jackson MD. Now or later? Attentional processing and intertemporal choice. J Behav Decis Mak 2016;29(2–3): 206–17.

23. Bond SM, Dietrich MS, Gilbert J, et al. Neurocognitive function in patients with head and neck cancer undergoing primary or adjuvant chemoradiation treatment. Support Care Cancer 2016; 24(10):4433–42.

24. Andreotti C, Root JC, Ahles TA, et al. Cancer, coping, and cognition: a model for the role of stress reactivity in cancer-related cognitive decline. Psychooncology 2015;24(6):617–23.

25. Silvers J, Buhle JT, Ochsner KN. The neuroscience of emotion regulation: basic mechanisms and their role in development, aging, and psychopathology. In: The oxford handbook of cognitive neuroscience: volume 2: the cutting edges. New York: Oxford University Press; 2013. Available at: http://www.oxfordhandbooks.com/view/10.1093/oxfordhb/9780199988709.001.0001/oxfordhb-9780199988709-e-026. Accessed January 20, 2018.

26. Hoesli RC, Shuman AG, Bradford CR. Decision making for diagnosis and management: a consensus comes to life. Otolaryngol Clin North Am 2017; 50(4):783–92.

27. Glajchen M. The emerging role and needs of family caregivers in cancer care. J Support Oncol 2004; 2(2):145–55.

28. Juster RP, Pruessner JC, Desrochers AB, et al. Sex and gender roles in relation to mental health and allostatic load. Psychosom Med 2016;78(7): 788–804.

29. Stacey D, Légaré F, Lewis K, et al. Decision aids for people facing health treatment or screening decisions. Cochrane Database Syst Rev 2017;(4): CD001431.

30. Cooper Z, Hevelone N, Sarhan M, et al. Identifying patient characteristics associated with deficits in surgical decision making. J Patient Saf 2016. [Epub ahead of print].

31. Lydiatt DD. Medical malpractice and head and neck cancer. Curr Opin Otolaryngol Head Neck Surg 2004;12(2):71–5.

32. Aaronson NK, Mattioli V, Minton O, et al. Beyond treatment - psychosocial and behavioural issues in cancer survivorship research and practice. EJC Suppl 2014;12(1):54–64.

33. Prochaska JO, Velicer WF. The transtheoretical model of health behavior change. Am J Health Promot 1997;12(1):38–48.

34. Henry M, Bdira A, Cherba M, et al. Recovering function and surviving treatments are primary motivators for health behavior change in patients with head and neck cancer: qualitative focus group study. Palliat Support Care 2016;14(4):364–75.

35. McCarter K, Martinez U, Britton B, et al. Smoking cessation care among patients with head and neck cancer: a systematic review. BMJ Open 2016;6(9): e012296.

36. Klimas J, Field C-A, Cullen W, et al. Psychosocial interventions to reduce alcohol consumption in concurrent problem alcohol and illicit drug users: Cochrane review. Syst Rev 2013;2:3.

37. Shields PG, Herbst RS, Arenberg D, et al. Smoking cessation, version 1.2016, NCCN clinical practice guidelines in oncology. J Natl Compr Canc Netw 2016;14(11):1430–68.

38. Kwon JH, Tanco K, Park JC, et al. Frequency, predictors, and medical record documentation of chemical coping among advanced cancer patients. Oncologist 2015;20(6):692–7.

39. Lawlor P, Walker P, Bruera E, et al. Severe opioid toxicity and somatization of psychosocial distress in a cancer patient with a background of chemical dependence. J Pain Symptom Manage 1997;13(6): 356–61.

40. Tawa. Overview of the genetics of alcohol use disorder. Alcohol Alcohol 2016;51(5):507–14.

41. Jamal N, Ebersole B, Erman A, et al. Maximizing functional outcomes in head and neck cancer survivors: assessment and rehabilitation. Otolaryngol Clin North Am 2017;50(4):837–52.

42. Steiner WA, Ryser L, Huber E, et al. Use of the ICF model as a clinical problem-solving tool in physical therapy and rehabilitation medicine. Phys Ther 2002;82(11):1098–107.

43. Kisser U, Adderson-Kisser C, Coenen M, et al. The development of an ICF-based clinical guideline and screening tool for the standardized assessment and evaluation of functioning after head and neck cancer treatment. Eur Arch Otorhinolaryngol 2017; 274(2).1035–43.

44. Henry M, Habib LA, Morrison M, et al. Head and neck cancer patients want us to support them psychologically in the post-treatment period: Survey results. Palliative & Supportive Care 2014;12(6): 481–93.

45. Goepfert RP, Fuller CD, Gunn GB, et al. Symptom burden as a driver of decisional regret in long-term oropharyngeal carcinoma survivors. Head Neck 2017;39(11):2151–8.

46. Pérez MMB, Menear M, Brehaut JC, et al. Extent and predictors of decision regret about health care decisions: a systematic review. Med Decis Mak 2016; 36(6):777–90.

47. Roussi. Monitoring style of coping with cancer related threats: a review of the literature. J Behav Med 2014;37(5):931–54.

48. Miller SM, Diefenbach MA. The Cognitive-Social Health Information-Processing (C-SHIP) model: a theoretical framework for research in behavioral oncology. Technology Methods Behav Med 1998; 219–44.

49. Macfarlane TV, Wirth T, Ranasinghe S, et al. Head and neck cancer pain: systematic review of prevalence and associated factors. J Oral Maxillofac Res 2012;3(1):e1.

50. Ripamonti CI, Santini D, Maranzano E, et al. Management of cancer pain: ESMO clinical practice guidelines. Ann Oncol 2012;23(Suppl 7):vii139–54.

51. Malfliet A, Coppieters I, Van Wilgen P, et al. Brain changes associated with cognitive and emotional factors in chronic pain: a systematic review. Eur J Pain 2017;21(5):769–86.

52. Terkawi AS, Tsang S, Alshehri AS, et al. The burden of chronic pain after major head and neck tumor therapy. Saudi J Anaesth 2017;11(Suppl 1):S71–9.

53. McMenamin EM, Grant M. Pain prevention using head and neck cancer as a model. J Adv Pract Oncol 2015;6(1):44–9.

54. Syrjala KL, Jensen MP, Mendoza ME, et al. Psychological and behavioral approaches to cancer pain management. J Clin Oncol 2014;32(16): 1703–11.

55. Mishra SI, Scherer RW, Snyder C, et al. Exercise interventions on health-related quality of life for people with cancer during active treatment. Cochrane Database Syst Rev 2012;(8):CD008465.

56. Sammut L, Ward M, Patel N. Physical activity and quality of life in head and neck cancer survivors: a literature review. Int J Sports Med 2014;35(9):794–9.

57. Hernandez Blazquez M, Cruzado JA. A longitudinal study on anxiety, depressive and adjustment disorder, suicide ideation and symptoms of emotional distress in patients with cancer undergoing radiotherapy. J Psychosom Res 2016;87:14–21.

58. Ghazali N, Cadwallader E, Lowe D, et al. Fear of recurrence among head and neck cancer survivors: longitudinal trends. Psycho-Oncology 2013;22(4): 807–13.

59. Abbey G, Thompson SB, Hickish T, et al. A meta-analysis of prevalence rates and moderating factors for cancer-related post-traumatic stress disorder. Psychooncology 2015;24(4):371–81.

60. Bisson JI, Roberts NP, Andrew M, et al. Psychological therapies for chronic post-traumatic stress disorder (PTSD) in adults. Cochrane Database Syst Rev 2013;(12):CD003388.

61. Rhoten BA. Head and neck cancer and sexuality: a review of the literature. Cancer Nurs 2016;39(4): 313–20.

62. Vehling S, Kissane DW, Lo C, et al. The association of demoralization with mental disorders and suicidal ideation in patients with cancer. Cancer 2017; 123(17):3394–401.

63. Barber B, Dergousoff J, Slater L, et al. Depression and survival in patients with head and neck cancer: a systematic review. JAMA Otolaryngol Head Neck Surg 2016;142(3):284–8.

64. Osazuwa-Peters N, Boakye EA, Mohammed KA, et al. Prevalence and sociodemographic predictors of depression in patients with head and neck cancer - results from a national study. J Clin Oncol 2016; 34(15_suppl):6064.

65. Robinson S, Kissane DW, Brooker J, et al. The relationship between poor quality of life and desire to hasten death: a multiple mediation model examining the contributions of depression, demoralization, loss of control, and low self-worth. J Pain Symptom Manage 2017;53(2):243–9.

66. Feen Ronjom M. Radiation-induced hypothyroidism after treatment of head and neck cancer. Dan Med J 2016;63(3) [pii:B5213].

67. Lydiatt WM, Moran J, Burke WJ. A review of depression in the head and neck cancer patient. Clin Adv Hematol Oncol 2009;7(6):397–403.

68. Newby JM, McKinnon A, Kuyken W, et al. Systematic review and meta-analysis of transdiagnostic psychological treatments for anxiety and depressive disorders in adulthood. Clin Psychol Rev 2015;40:91–110.

69. Henry M, Rosberger Z, Ianovski LE, et al. A screening algorithm for early detection of major depressive disorder in head and neck cancer patients post-treatment: Longitudinal study. Psychooncology 2018;27(6):1622–8.

70. De Boer MF, McCormick LK, Pruyn JF, et al. Physical and psychosocial correlates of head and neck cancer: a review of the literature. Otolaryngol Head Neck Surg 1999;120(3):427–36.

71. Rieke K, Schmid KK, Lydiatt W, et al. Depression and survival in head and neck cancer patients. Oral Oncol 2017;65:76–82.

72. Rapee RM, Heimberg RG. A cognitive-behavioral model of anxiety in social phobia. Behav Res Ther 1997;35(8):741–56.

73. Henry M. Looking beyond disfigurement: the experience of patients with head and neck cancer. J Palliat Care 2014;30(1):5–15.

74. Cash TF, Smolak L. Body image: a handbook of science, practice, and prevention. New York: Guilford Press; 2011.

75. Fingeret MC, Teo I, Epner DE. Managing body image difficulties of adult cancer patients: lessons from available research. Cancer 2014; 120(5):633–41.

76. Rhoten BA. Body image disturbance in adults treated for cancer - a concept analysis. J Adv Nurs 2016;72(5):1001–11.

77. Henry M, Alias A. Body image and functional loss. In: Fingeret MC, Teo I, editors. Principles and Practices of Body Image Care For Cancer Patients. New York: Oxford University Press; 2018.

78. White CA. Body image dimensions and cancer: a heuristic cognitive behavioural model. Psychooncology 2000;9(3):183–92.

79. Scott DW, Oberst MT, Dropkin MJ. A stress-coping model. ANS Adv Nurs Sci 1980;3(1):9–23.

80. Bultz BD, Cummings GG, Grassi L, et al. 2013 President's Plenary International Psycho-oncology Society: embracing the IPOS standards as a means of enhancing comprehensive cancer care. Psychooncology 2014;23(9):1073–8.

81. Krebber AM, Jansen F, Witte BI, et al. Stepped care targeting psychological distress in head and neck cancer and lung cancer patients: a randomized, controlled trial. Ann Oncol 2016;27(9):1754–60.

82. Henry M, Rosberger Z, Bertrand L, et al. Prevalence and Risk Factors of Suicidal Ideation among Patients with Head and Neck Cancer: Longitudinal Study. Otolaryngol Head Neck Surg 2018.

Printed and bound by CPI Group (UK) Ltd, Croydon, CR0 4YY

08/05/2025

01864734-0002